Caring for
Loved Ones with
HEART
DISEASE

Caring for
Loved Ones with
HEART
DISEASE

J SHAH, MD

ROWMAN & LITTLEFIELD
Lanham • Boulder • New York • London

This book represents reference material only. It is not intended as a medical manual, and the data presented here are meant to assist the reader in making informed choices regarding health. This book is not a replacement for treatment(s) that the reader's personal physician may have suggested. If the reader believes he or she is experiencing a medical issue, professional medical help is recommended. Mention of particular products, companies, or authorities in this book does not entail endorsement by the publisher or author.

Published by Rowman & Littlefield
An imprint of The Rowman & Littlefield Publishing Group, Inc.
4501 Forbes Boulevard, Suite 200, Lanham, Maryland 20706
www.rowman.com

86-90 Paul Street, London EC2A 4NE, United Kingdom

British Library Cataloguing in Publication Information on file

Library of Congress Cataloging-in-Publication Data
Names: Shah, J, 1973– author.
Title: Caring for loved ones with heart disease / J Shah, MD.
Description: Lanham : Rowman & Littlefield, 2022. | Includes bibliographical
   references and index.
Identifiers: LCCN 2021040418 (print) | LCCN 2021040419 (ebook) |
   ISBN 9781538162323 (cloth) | ISBN 9781538162330 (epub)
Subjects: LCSH: Heart—Diseases—Patients. | Heart—Diseases—Patients—Care.
Classification: LCC RC682 .S43 2022 (print) | LCC RC682 (ebook) |
   DDC 362.1/9612—dc23
LC record available at https://lccn.loc.gov/2021040418
LC ebook record available at https://lccn.loc.gov/2021040419

This book is dedicated to the millions of family members, friends, neighbors, and professionals who provide care and support to people with heart disease.

CONTENTS

HOW TO USE THIS BOOK

This book is intended for caregivers whose loved ones have been diagnosed with heart disease. It is written for readers with all levels of familiarity with heart disease and the related tests and treatments. *Caring for Loved Ones with Heart Disease* contains a series of questions that caregivers most commonly have while looking after their loved ones. If you have a question, it is likely that others in your situation have had the same question and is included in this book along with answers.

It is recommended that you begin by familiarizing yourself with each section of the book. Reading and understanding chapter 1 will help you familiarize yourself with terms that your health care team will use frequently. The figures provided will give you a visual reference that will be useful throughout this journey.

Chapter 2 will help the caregiver understand the various symptoms of heart disease, what these symptoms indicate, and how to work with the health care team to improve these symptoms. Chapter 5 will build upon this by explaining various heart conditions as well as tests and treatments that a heart patient may undergo. You can use the above chapters to get better acquainted with the language as well as the process of care in heart disease. By learning about this beforehand, you will understand the information that the health care team will provide and be able participate in the decision-making process. It will also help you take better care of the person before and after heart-related tests and procedures.

Chapter 3 addresses the critical issue of taking care of yourself on this long journey with your loved one. It will provide you with tools to organize and coordinate the care of your loved one so as to provide best care for him or her while caring for yourself.

Chapter 4 discusses the delicate conversation regarding goals of care including end-of-life care for your loved ones. It provides you with tips and tools for getting paperwork in order so that the treatment path follows the wishes of the person rather than the vagaries of the system.

Chapter 6 addresses the subjects of exercise, diet, and weight-related issues in heart disease. It will equip you with pertinent information that may not be discussed adequately at the doctor's office. The chapter will also guide you to ensure physical and emotional safety of your loved one.

Medications are the cornerstone of care for patients with heart disease. Safe and appropriate use of medicines will increase the life span of many patients with heart disease, but medication error could create a dangerous situation. Chapter 7 offers you an overview of medication management and medication safety. It further offers you the answers to many questions regarding specific medicines used in heart disease.

Your health care team will have many members from various settings including clinics, hospitals, and other locations. Each member will have specialized knowledge in their field. Knowing their expertise and roles, as described in chapter 8, will help you seek out the right expert for the questions that you may have. This will decrease the frustration that many caregivers endure trying to get answers they need to provide care to their loved ones. It will also give you an opinion from a true expert in that field.

Chapter 9 provides worksheets to help you gather the information a caregiver needs to have on hand so as to facilitate seamless care through an otherwise fragmented health care system.

Some chapters will be relevant to your situation now, while others may inform future situations and decisions. You may decide to read cover to cover, or you may skip around according to your current needs. Research has found that people who use resources like this book or other information material are more confident in handling medical issues.

When you encounter a new problem, be sure to check the book for guidance. For problems you encounter often, review the relevant section of this book and bookmark pages for reference.

You may also find it useful to review sections of the book for potential problems that may occur. Some readers may want to review the information in chapter 1 before visiting a health care provider to refamiliarize themselves with the heart and its workings. All of this is a good way to increase your confidence and be prepared for the current and possible future situations. The successful use of this book will be indicated by bookmarks and sticky notes you scatter through various sections of this book for ready reference. More enthusiastic readers may personalize it by adding their own notes on the sides.

The recording sheets and checklists can be photocopied or torn out for use. Remember to have them handy when you communicate with health care providers.

Some of the information in the book may appear repetitious. It is partly done to highlight and stress the important information and partly to enable readers who read selective sections to still have a complete grasp of the necessary information. Hopefully, you will find that this strategy leads to better understanding of material covered, regardless of the way in which you decide to use this book.

ACKNOWLEDGMENTS

This book, as all endeavors of an individual, is a team effort. My team included patients; their family members; nurses, nurse practitioners, and doctors specializing in heart conditions; and case managers and social workers in many hospitals I have had the privilege to work in. I am especially grateful for my family and friends who have made me the person I have become and the doctor I yearn to be day after day.

First and foremost, I am grateful to the heart failure staff at Essentia Health, namely Dr. Kimberly Boddicker, Linda Wick, Denise Buxbaum, Michelle Anderson, and Lynne Bergal, for contributing to this book by sharing their immense knowledge and experiences with patients and caregivers. Denise, Lynne, and Michelle took precious time out of their personal lives to review several chapters of this book. I am grateful for their detailed review.

Michael Petty, a nurse practitioner at University of Minnesota, guided me through his decades of experience with patients and caregivers. He provided me with insights for the caregivers, which many loved ones may only learn after considerable turmoil.

My brother, Ketan, has been by my side through the thick and thin of my life and has supported me in good times and bad, in my exhilarations and frustrations, success and failures, without judging, prodding, or blaming but always encouraging and cheering. He reviewed every chapter with the detail that only a brother would, despite battling several competing priorities. My girlfriend, Rebecca, who I ignored for many months while I spent time working on the book, reviewed every chapter, making suggestions in her gentle way, and the final product is much better because of her input. I am extremely grateful for Chetan Kasargod, MD, who went through the book with a fine-tooth comb and made important suggestions regarding details, styles, and wordings. His conversations with thousands of patients and caregivers are reflected in this book. My friend, philosopher, and guide Dennis Menezes, who has believed in my ability to write despite occasional evidence to the contrary, has continued to be a source of guidance when I was lost in a mountain of information without a clear way to convey it. None of my writing would be possible without his encouragement and wisdom.

I am grateful to Mary Van Beusekom, who suffered through my many spelling and grammatical errors in early drafts and helped in editing this book to make it readable for all. I am indebted to Lauren Whale, who continues to make herself available for editorial assistance, despite her many competing priorities. I am grateful to my agent, Anne Devlin, and my publisher, Rowman & Littlefield, and their editorial staff for making this book a reality.

FOREWORD

The health care system is complex even for people who work in health care. Navigating the system as a patient or caregiver can be overwhelming. A caregiver is often emotionally taxed every step of the way when helping a loved one navigate the system, in addition to providing care. This book offers practical advice and tools for the caregiver of patients with chronic heart disease. It is a beacon of light in the dark for caregivers.

I have been a nurse practitioner for almost thirty years, specifically dealing with chronic heart failure patients. I currently serve as president of the American Association of Heart Failure Nurses (AAHFN). The information in this book is something I've wanted for caregivers, but it has not been available. There is a plethora of patient education, caregiver tools, and guides on the market. However, it is not all in one place. There is not one reference guide that covers the journey of advanced heart disease. Like our health care system, the information available has many gaps. As an NP, I know I have to keep instructions simple for the caregivers, as they are often not health care professionals and absorbing a lot of information at once will not happen. So we end up giving them bits of information at a time—how to manage symptoms, information on medications, and so forth. Often the handouts are lost between visits, and what we don't have is a guide on how to navigate the health care system. Having all this information, presented in a simple format, in one reference guide is what has been missing in my practice.

There is a great need for this book as it will serve as a reference for caregivers as they travel this journey with their loved one. It provides references to other resources if needed but gives the basics for caregivers. We know if caregivers are empowered and informed, the patient does better. The end result is providing better patient care, which equates to better outcomes. This book will be welcomed by clinicians as well as patients and caregivers.

The author of this book, Dr. J Shah, brings a perspective that highlights his global training and experience of health care delivery. Given his atypical background in epidemiology, biostatistics, medicine, cardiology, and electrophysiology and as a researcher and now published author, his expertise from multiple disciplines is woven into the fabric of this book. Dr. Shah has lived in many different locations and cultures in the world. I believe this worldview experience has molded his values about the importance of family caregivers of patients with heart disease. Although the culture the patient lives in may differ, this book crosses that cultural barrier and focuses on what all heart patients and their caregivers need to know.

—Linda Wick, President
American Association of Heart Failure Nurses (AAHFN)

One

THE BASICS

I didn't understand a lot. I wish someone would explain it to me in simple language. I feel that once I read about how the heart works, I will be able to grapple with what the doctor said.
—*Terri, daughter of a person with heart disease*

Being the caregiver of a person with heart disease is an important and immense responsibility. It involves caring for the person at home and participating in health care decisions in clinics and hospitals. In order to feel equipped for these responsibilities, it is critical to understand the heart, its normal functioning, and common diseases affecting it. Such an understanding will help you make informed choices about the person's care at home and interact meaningfully with the health care team.

SECTION 1: BASICS OF THE HEART: WHAT DOES THE HEART DO?

The heart is a fist-sized, muscular organ to the left of center in the chest. Each minute, the heart beats sixty to one hundred times and pumps five liters of oxygen-rich blood. The oxygen is used by other organs in the body and returned to the heart.

The Four Chambers of the Heart (figure 1.1)

- **Right atrium:** The upper chamber, the right atrium, receives oxygen-poor blood from the body and pushes it through the tricuspid valve into the right bottom chamber, or right ventricle.
- **Right ventricle:** This heart chamber receives oxygen-poor blood from the right atrium and pumps it via the pulmonary valve into the lungs. In the lungs, the blood picks up oxygen and flows through the pulmonary veins into the left upper chamber, or left atrium.

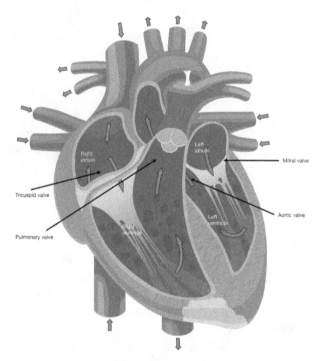

Figure 1.1. There are four chambers in the heart: the right atrium, right ventricle, left atrium, and left ventricle. The heart's four valves consist of the tricuspid valve, pulmonary valve, mitral valve, and aortic valve.
© *iStock/Getty Images Plus/melazerg*

- **Left atrium:** The left atrium receives blood from the lungs and passes it through the mitral valve into the left lower chamber, or left ventricle.
- **Left ventricle:** This heart chamber receives oxygen-rich blood from the left atrium. Once the left ventricle is filled, its powerful muscles squeeze (contract) and push the blood through the aortic valve to the aorta and the rest of the body.

The Heart's Four Valves

- **Tricuspid valve:** Allows blood to go in one direction, from the right atrium to the right ventricle.
- **Pulmonary valve:** Allows blood to go in one direction, from the right ventricle to the arteries to the lungs.
- **Mitral valve:** Allows blood to go in one direction, from the left atrium to the left ventricle.
- **Aortic valve:** Allows blood to go in one direction, from the left ventricle to the aorta.

In addition to chambers and valves, the heart has muscles that contract and expel blood. This muscle action of the left ventricle provides blood to the body.

The next critical structures to understand are the arteries, which supply oxygen-rich blood to the heart muscles so they function efficiently. These arteries are called coronary arteries (figure 1.2).

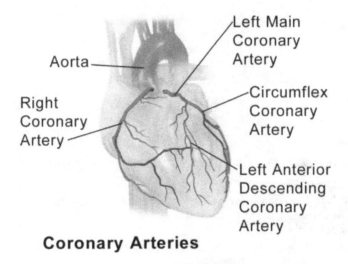

Coronary Arteries

Figure 1.2. There are two coronary arteries, the right and the left. The left main coronary artery further divides into the left anterior descending artery and the left circumflex artery. © *Wikimedia Commons/Bruce Blaus*

There are two coronary arteries, the right and the left. The left main coronary artery further divides into the left anterior descending artery and the left circumflex artery.

The final piece of the heart puzzle is the electrical system of the heart (figure 1.3).

The heart's spark plug is the sinoatrial node. This node, located in the right upper chamber, starts a normal heartbeat. From here, the electrical activity spreads to the two upper chambers and then to the atrioventricular junction, a bridge between the upper and lower chambers. After a minor delay on this bridge, the electricity spreads to the lower chamber. The spread of the electrical signal then initiates mechanical contraction of the heart chambers. In a normal heart, the upper chambers get the electrical signal and contract first. Moments later, the lower chamber receives the electrical impulses and contracts. The upper and lower chambers contract (beat) one

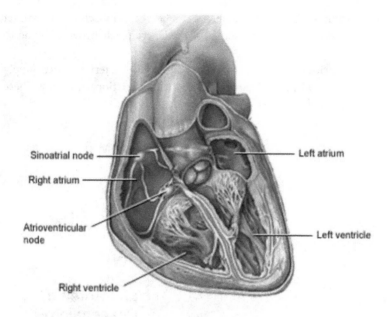

Sinoatrial node

Right atrium

Atrioventricular node

Right ventricle

Left atrium

Left ventricle

Figure 1.3. The heart's electrical system provides the electrical spark to start the squeezing action of the muscles. *MedlinePlus from the National Library of Medicine*

after another in a rhythmic, coordinated manner sixty to one hundred times a minute (hence the corresponding pulse rate of sixty to one hundred a minute).

In summary, these are the four components of the heart:

- the muscles that contract blood to the body and perform the pumping function of the heart,
- the valves that ensure blood flow in the correct direction,
- the coronary arteries that carry oxygen-rich blood to nourish the heart muscle, and
- an electrical system that provides the electrical spark to start the squeezing action of the muscles.

WHAT IS CORONARY ARTERY DISEASE?

Coronary artery disease is a condition in which one or more of the three major arteries that supply blood to the heart muscle get narrow. This decreases the blood supply to the heart muscle. If there is a sudden and complete blockage in the blood flow in a coronary artery, it causes heart attack (myocardial infarction).

WHAT IS CARDIAC ARREST?

Cardiac arrest is an emergency condition in which the heart stops pumping blood altogether. A person suffering from cardiac arrest will have difficulty breathing and then will lose consciousness and collapse within seconds. Unless action is taken within seconds to minutes, cardiac arrest can be fatal. CPR performed in time while waiting for emergency services to arrive may save the life of a person having cardiac arrest.

Heart attack can cause cardiac arrest, but cardiac arrest can also occur from electrical problems of the heart.

WHAT IS HEART FAILURE?

Heart failure is a condition in which the heart muscle is weak and does not work normally. It cannot provide enough oxygen-rich blood to the body. Occasionally, heart failure can also be caused by heart muscle stiffness.

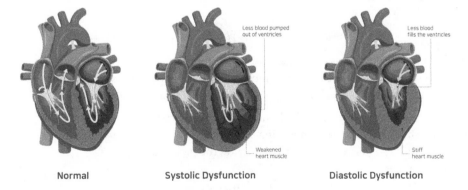

Normal   Systolic Dysfunction   Diastolic Dysfunction

Figure 1.4. Left: normal heart; center: heart failure from weak heart; right: heart failure from stiff heart. © iStock/Getty Images Plus/go-un lee

WHAT CAUSES WEAKNESS OF THE HEART MUSCLE?

Weakness of the heart muscle, known as cardiomyopathy, can be caused by many conditions:

- one or more heart attacks,
- damaged heart valves (e.g., leaky or blocked heart valves),
- a virus affecting heart muscles,
- long-term untreated high blood pressure,
- untreated rapid heartbeats for weeks,
- alcohol abuse,
- drug abuse,
- cancer-related medicines,
- other conditions affecting heart muscles (e.g., hypertrophic cardiomyopathy),
- severe lung disease, and
- inflammation of the heart muscle, or myocarditis.

WHAT ARE THE EFFECTS OF HEART FAILURE?

In heart failure, the heart does not pump enough oxygen-rich blood to the body. The organs do not get the required blood supply. Kidneys react to this by retaining water and salt in the body. This results in fluid buildup in the legs and ankles, causing them to swell. Fluid buildup in the lungs interferes with breathing, causing shortness of breath. If untreated, heart failure causes the heart valves to leak and abnormal rhythm problems in the electrical system. Over time, other body organs are damaged due to lack of oxygen.

WHAT ARE THE SYMPTOMS OF HEART FAILURE?

In the early stages, people may not have symptoms, but over the years, they develop one or more of these symptoms. Often, people dismiss these symptoms as a normal part of aging. You should be vigilant for these symptoms:

- shortness of breath with physical activity or at rest;
- shortness of breath while lying flat in bed;
- sudden shortness of breath that wakes the person at night;
- fatigue;
- dry, hacking cough or cough with mucus;
- swelling of the ankles and legs;
- poor appetite and nausea;
- bloating of the abdomen.

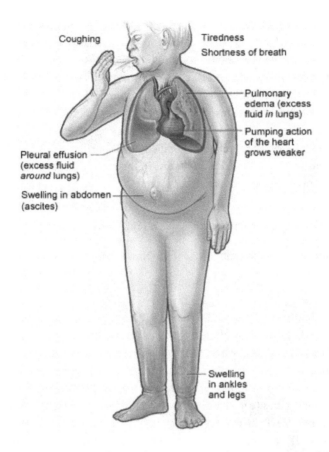

Coughing

Tiredness
Shortness of breath

Pulmonary edema (excess fluid *in* lungs)

Pumping action of the heart grows weaker

Pleural effusion (excess fluid *around* lungs)

Swelling in abdomen (ascites)

Swelling in ankles and legs

Figure 1.5. Symptoms of heart failure. *National Heart, Lung, and Blood Institute, National Institutes of Health, US Department of Health and Human Services*

WHAT ARE THE COMPLICATIONS OF HEART FAILURE?

- **Organ damage:** Low blood flow to the body can interfere with the function of various organs. The kidneys are most susceptible due to low blood flow. People with advanced heart failure can have kidney failure and need dialysis.
- **Fluid buildup in the liver:** When the heart is weak and cannot pump blood efficiently, it can build up in the lungs and gradually flow back and accumulate in the liver. Over time, this can put pressure on the liver and affect liver function.

- **Fluid buildup in the stomach and intestines:** This makes them soggy. A person may notice a decrease in appetite and change in bowel habits.
- **Enlargement of the heart:** Heart failure can cause enlargement of the heart. In an enlarged heart, the valves may not work properly. Heart valve problems (e.g., mitral regurgitation) may occur.
- **Abnormal heart rhythms:** With the enlargement of the chambers of the heart and valve leaks, people with heart failure can develop heart rhythm problems in the upper chamber, called atrial fibrillation. They can also have ominous heart rhythm problems in the lower chamber, like ventricular tachycardia/ventricular fibrillation.

HOW DO WE KNOW WHEN HEART FAILURE IS WORSENING?

Heart failure is classified into one of four classes based on symptoms:

- **Class I:** The person has no symptoms and can carry out all activities without any problems.
- **Class II:** The person has little to no limitation in performing day-to-day activities (e.g., dressing, going to the bathroom, showering). However, he gets tired and winded when climbing a couple flights of stairs or walking uphill.
- **Class III:** The person has marked limitation in performing normal activities. Activities (e.g., dressing, making the bed, going to the bathroom, showering) leave the person tired or out of breath.
- **Class IV:** The person is uncomfortable, tired, and winded even at rest.

The goal is to keep people in Class I and II using treatment at home so they can enjoy everyday activities and have a normal life. When people get to Class III, they may need hospitalization or more aggressive treatment at home to prevent advancing to Class IV and, hopefully, revert to Class II. People with Class IV need hospitalization for intravenous medicine and other treatments.

HOW IS HEART FAILURE DIAGNOSED?

Doctors diagnose heart failure if the person has the symptoms mentioned previously and a weak heart on echocardiography.

Doctors use echocardiography to check the pumping capacity of the heart. Pumping function is expressed as a number called ejection fraction.

In simpler words, if the left bottom chamber of the heart (called the left ventricle) receives 100 milliliters of blood and pumps out or *ejects* 60 milliliters, the ejection fraction is 60 percent in this case. A normal heart has an ejection fraction of 55 percent or more. People with heart failure have lower ejection fractions (i.e., less than 40 percent).

An echocardiogram can also help the doctor detect if the heart muscles are stiff rather than weak, a condition called diastolic heart failure. This test also informs the doctor about the possible causes of heart failure (e.g., previous heart attacks, heart valve problems, untreated high blood pressure).

Electrocardiography, a stress test, cardiac catheterization, blood tests, chest radiograph, or magnetic resonance imaging may be performed to detect other causes of heart failure. In rare instances, a heart biopsy is recommended.

SECTION 2: BASICS OF CAREGIVING: THE ROLE OF CAREGIVERS

"It takes a village to care for a person with advanced heart disease" may sound like a cliché. However, this paradigm can guide you in ensuring a long and healthy life for your loved one despite advanced heart disease.

This village includes two teams: the health care team and the home care team. The health care team includes the person, you as the caregiver, doctors, nurse practitioners, nurses, pharmacists, physical and occupational therapists, social workers, and counselors.

The home care team consists of you, the person, family and friends, home health aides, and home health nurses. The teams work together to offer continuity between the person's home and clinics and hospitals. As you may notice, you and the person form the link between the two teams; you are critical to ensuring the seamless transition from one setting to another and navigating the health care system effectively and efficiently.

Due to the natural course of heart disease, people go through phases of being at home alternating with occasional visits to the clinic intermingled with short and long hospitalizations. You also have a varied role throughout these different phases.

Depending on the phase, you may sometimes play a large role on the team, while the person may take control at other times. You will oversee all aspects of home care and elements of health care to help the person enjoy many years with a high quality of life.

You are the most important team member for a person with advanced heart disease. You can provide physical, intellectual, emotional, and spiritual support and be a friend, nurse, assistant, and spokesperson by understanding:

- the person: his priorities, likes, and dislikes;
- the health condition: symptoms and treatment options and plans; and
- other team members: their roles and responsibilities.

Most caregivers are spouses or offspring and so usually know the person for years before his diagnosis of heart disease. They know the person's priorities, likes and dislikes, dietary preferences, his tolerance for different forms of exercise, and temperament.

If you understand the recommended diet, you can prepare it according to the person's preferences. You may act as a coach and encourage the person to be physically active per the recommendations. You may join in the physical activity, making it a social event while also monitoring the person's symptoms during these activities. You may further act as a cheerleader to foster a sense of accomplishment with each success, no matter how big or small.

By knowing the person's disposition and recognizing the impact of the disease on his mental health, you can recognize emotional changes early and facilitate their early treatment.

Although you may know the person well, the disease takes its toll and may change the person's preferences. For example, an otherwise active, healthy person who was "always on the move" may prefer to be in bed for hours due to heart disease–related lethargy, side effects of medicines, or depression. Hence, understanding the disease and its physical and emotional implications helps you meet the person's needs.

Heart failure is a chronic disease with intermittent hospitalizations. However, most people and caregivers prefer to recover at home rather than in the hospital. Understanding the disease, its course, early signs of the need for hospitalization, and possible treatment options at home will help you in the role as nurse. You monitor changes in diet, weight, blood pressure, and medicine use. Early recognition of any changes and a timely call to the doctor's office or visit to the clinic may prevent hospitalizations.

While talking to the doctor's office or during the clinic visit, you can be an effective advocate and spokesperson for the person. During clinic visits, tests and treatments are recommended, and medicines are adjusted. The person may be too tired or stressed to ask the appropriate questions if the doctor recommends surgery or medicine. You act as an extra set of eyes, pair of ears, and brain to help the person process the information and ensure that the tests and treatments are in keeping with the person's priorities.

When the person undergoes tests, treatments, and procedures throughout the course of his disease, you ensure a smooth transition from home to the hospital and back again. You can help the person prepare for tests and treatments. While the person is in the hospital, you can give the health care team the information they need. You also receive and help carry out the instructions these team members give about the person's care.

Back at home, with a good understanding of these tests and treatments, you once again nurse the person back to health. Later in the course of the disease, if the person cannot speak for himself, you speak for him to ensure that his wishes and preferences are respected at the end of his life.

Caregiving is a tough job with physical, emotional, and financial effects. Two-thirds of caregivers have increased stress, and half of them skip their own doctors' appointments. Furthermore, about two-thirds of caregivers have financial worries that arise due to caregiving. All of this can lead to caregiver burnout. However, burnout has been underrecognized despite its negative effect on you and the person.

Self-care involving adequate sleep, a nutritious diet, and regular exercise helps, but a support system is also needed. Recently, steps have been identified to prevent and combat burnout. Several resources can provide emotional and social support and a much-needed respite from caregiving. Being aware of local and statewide support systems and services helps you feel equipped for your pivotal role in the person's care.

RESOURCES FOR HELP

Caring for someone with advanced heart disease can be physically and emotionally draining. This book covers many of the key issues. There are many other helpful resources as well.

The person's health care provider is a good place to start in finding resources. In addition, every county or region in the country has organizations that can provide guidance, such as the American Heart Association and the American Association of Heart Failure Nurses.

Support groups in most communities help caregivers compare notes with others having similar experiences. Here are some more resources:

Communications Tips for Caregivers

- American Heart Association EmPOWERED to Serve (empoweredtoserve .org/en/health-topics/caregiver-support/communication-tips-for-care givers): Find information and tips on communicating with family members and the health care team.

Emotional Support

- American Heart Association Caregiver Message Board (supportnetwork .heart.org/connect-with-people-like-me/caregiver/caregiver-heart/): Communicate with other caregivers and ask questions.
- Caregiver Action Network (855-227-3640; caregiveraction.org/resources): Find education, peer support, and resources.
- Mended Hearts (mendedhearts.org/): Find online support, lectures, and conferences.
- Next Step in Care (nextstepincare.org): Find information on enabling smooth care transitions.
- The Family Caregiver Alliance (caregiver.org): Find information and connect with other caregivers.

Information

- American Association of Heart Failure Nurses (https://www.aahfn.org/ mpage/patient_tip_sheet): Find advice on diet, exercise, medications, and so forth. Resources for patient and caregiver empowerment are also available.
- Aging Care (agingcare.com/topics/81/heart-disease/articles): Find a library of articles on common issues facing caregivers of people with heart disease.
- Care.com (care.com/senior-care-caring-for-seniors-with-heart-disease -p1143-q317306.html): Find advice, a question-and-answer section, and information on caring for someone with heart disease.

Respite Care

- Area Agency on Aging (payingforseniorcare.com/longtermcare/find_ aging_agencies_adrc_aaa.html): Find information on nutrition, how to receive an in-home care assessment, care plan development, referrals to community-based assistance programs, and long-term care facilities and get assistance with insurance and transportation.
- Visiting Nurses of America (vnaa.org): Find local in-home nurses.

Two

MANAGING COMMON SYMPTOMS OF HEART DISEASE

Initially when she developed heart disease, I was scared and worried. I didn't know what to do when she was getting winded or had leg swelling. I would rush to the emergency room every time. Now I know a lot more and feel that I can handle most things at home under the doctor's guidance.

—Leonard, whose wife has heart disease

I n this chapter, we will discuss the how and why of various symptoms of heart disease such as chest pain, shortness of breath, palpitations, and syncope. You will get an overview of what you should do immediately and also what to expect from the health care providers when you tell them about these symptoms. Understanding these symptoms and the treatments offered will help you and the person overcome anxiety and navigate heart conditions with confidence.

CHEST PAIN

Chest pain is the most common and concerning symptom in people with heart disease. Depending on the circumstance, it can be benign or life threatening.

The person may describe the pain as burning, pressure, crushing pain, dull ache, or tightness in the chest or like an elephant is sitting on the chest. The pain may radiate to the jaw, neck, or shoulder. People may also have nausea or vomiting, cold sweats, lightheadedness, dizziness, or shortness of breath.

The chest pain may get worse with exercise and better with rest. Some people find relief by sitting up or lying down. Others notice that the pain worsens with coughing or deep breaths. In some cases, chest pain is accompanied by a sour taste in the mouth or trouble swallowing. Some people are able to cause the pain by pushing on the chest. Chest pain may last from a minute to hours. Caregivers can help the doctor make a diagnosis by paying attention to these details.

How Do Heart Problems Cause Chest Pain?

Chest pain can indicate a range of heart problems such as:

- heart attack: sudden and complete blockage in the coronary artery that cuts off the blood supply to the heart muscle;
- angina: decreased blood flow to the heart muscle due to narrowing of the heart artery; or
- inflammation (rare): an inflamed heart muscle (myocarditis) or sac surrounding the heart (pericarditis).

Chest pain can be caused by non-heart-related problems such as:

- aortic dissection: a torn aorta, a big blood vessel in the chest;
- reflux disease in the esophagus, the food pipe;
- ulcer in the stomach or inflammation of the stomach;
- inflammation or injury of the muscles, ribs, or cartilage of the breast bone;
- pneumonia;
- collapsed lungs;
- pleurisy: inflammation of the sac covering the lungs;
- pulmonary embolism: blood clot in the artery that supplies blood to the lungs;
- inflammation of the gallbladder or gallstones;
- inflammation of the pancreas; or
- panic and stress.

When Is Chest Pain Worrisome Enough to Call for Help?

Call 911 for any of the following symptoms:

- pain that starts suddenly and continues even when the person rests;
- chest pain in a person who has had a previous heart attack, bypass surgery, or recent stent placement;
- nausea, vomiting, dizziness, or lightheadedness along with chest pain; or
- new chest pain that lasts longer than a minute and does not resolve with nitroglycerin tablets.

Call the doctor's office if:

- the chest pain has been constant and ongoing for days;
- the chest pain is accompanied by swallowing problems; or
- the person had a fever or cough before the onset of chest pain.

When you call the doctor's office, be ready to answer the following questions:

- What is the person's name?
- What is the person's date of birth?
- Who is the person's primary cardiologist?
- Has the person had bypass surgery? Stents?
- When did the person last have a stress test or cardiac catheterization?
- Does the person have high blood pressure or diabetes?
- What medicines does the person use currently? Any over-the-counter medicines? Supplements?
- Any recent changes to the medicines?
- Has the person recently stopped taking any medicines?

When you go to the emergency department or doctor's office, be prepared to answer the following questions:

- When did the person's symptoms start?
- Describe the pain. Does it radiate to the jaw, neck, or shoulders? Does it worsen with exertion? Does it worsen with deep breaths? With cough? Has the pain gotten better or worse over time? Is the pain accompanied by nausea, cold sweats, lightheadedness, dizziness, or shortness of breath?
- Does the person have a heart condition?
- Does the person smoke? Did he smoke in the past? How much?
- Do any of the person's first-degree relatives have heart disease?
- Does the person have other health conditions (e.g., diabetes, high blood pressure, reflux disease, gallbladder problems)?
- Has the person traveled recently?
- Has the person been bedridden of late?
- Does the person use alcohol or caffeine? How much?
- Does the person use illegal medicines (e.g., cocaine)?
- Has the person had chest pain before? If so, what was the diagnosis?

What Tests Will the Doctor Likely Recommend?

- electrocardiogram (EKG): to look for evidence of a major heart attack;

- blood tests: to look for evidence of minor heart attacks not detected on an electrocardiogram or non-heart-related conditions;
- CT scan (computed tomography): to look for blood clots in the lungs or a torn aorta;
- chest X-ray: to look for pneumonia or collapsed lungs;
- stress test: to look for narrowing of the coronary arteries;
- cardiac catheterization: to look for blockages in the coronary arteries (this is performed if the electrocardiogram or blood tests suggest heart attack, the stress test is abnormal, or there is a strong suspicion of blockages in the coronary arteries); or
- echo (echocardiogram): to look at heart function, valve problems, or evidence of previous heart attacks.

What Treatment Options May Be Offered for Heart-Related Chest Pain?

- aspirin: this is the first medicine that people with chest pain usually receive in the emergency department;
- nitroglycerin, under the tongue or intravenous: for relief of chest pain;
- morphine, intravenous: for relief of chest pain that continues despite taking nitroglycerin;
- blood thinners: if heart attack or blood clots in the lungs are suspected;
- emergency angioplasty: for major heart attack;
- thrombolytics (clot-busting medicines): for major heart attack (as an alternative to emergency angioplasty); or
- emergency bypass surgery: for multiple blocked coronary arteries (in rare circumstances, after cardiac catheterization is performed and when angioplasty is not possible, this surgery may be recommended).

How Can I Help the Person in This Situation?

During the episode of chest pain, you can observe whether the person has nausea, dizziness, or shortness of breath or is getting close to passing out. You can note the duration of the chest pain and any associated pain in the arm, neck, or jaw. You can also note factors that make the pain better or worse. If the doctor has prescribed a medicine to be used during such episodes, you should give it to the person.

Based on the previously mentioned guidance, you should call 911 if needed. In the emergency department, you should help the person recall the details of the episode and bring the person's medical history and medicine list.

Before the person is released from the hospital, you should ask the following questions:

- Do we know what caused the chest pain? If not, what is the most likely cause? How serious is this condition?
- Does the person need to be hospitalized?
- What tests have been done?
- What is the treatment plan?
- Is the person going to see a specialist? When?
- If the person is released to home, what are the next steps?
- Are there any changes in the person's medicines?

If the doctor says that the chest pain is not cause for concern, you should remind the person of this and calm him during the next episode.

SHORTNESS OF BREATH

Doctors and nurses may call it shortness of breath, dyspnea, or shortness of air. People may feel smothered, tire easily, or have shortness of breath when walking stairs or doing simple day-to-day activities.

If a person ignores these symptoms, they may eventually be unable to lie flat while sleeping, need more pillows to raise their head, or wake at night feeling breathless. Some people may cough frequently and, in extreme situations, produce mucus or pink, blood-tinged sputum while coughing. Ongoing, constant chest pressure may also be associated with this condition.

You may notice that the person wheezes or that their breath is rapid and shallow—even before they complain. Some people ignore these symptoms or attribute their symptoms to another cause. Astute caregivers know that these symptoms indicate fluid retention in people with an advanced heart condition.

While shortness of breath may also be due to other conditions, people with a heart condition may have swelling of the feet, ankles, legs, or abdomen (ascites). They may also have subtle, nonspecific symptoms such as fatigue, decreased appetite, increased urination at night, nausea, or difficulty concentrating.

It is important to look for these symptoms and alert the person's health care providers so they can formulate a diagnosis.

Shortness of breath may be caused by heart conditions such as:

- coronary artery disease,
- heart failure,
- narrowing of a valve,
- uncontrolled high blood pressure, or
- valve leak.

Shortness of breath may also be caused by non-heart-related conditions such as pneumonia, emphysema, chronic obstructive pulmonary disease, anemia, and generalized weakness.

How Do Heart Problems Cause Shortness of Breath?

When the heart is weak, it cannot pump blood efficiently, which causes blood to back up into the veins in the lungs. This increases pressure and pushes fluid into the air spaces in the lungs, which can reduce the movement of oxygen through the lungs and cause shortness of breath.

When Is the Shortness of Breath Concerning Enough to Call the Doctor's Office?

If the person has any of the following symptoms, contact the doctor's office:

- shortness of breath at rest,
- new and unusual cough,
- progressive shortness of breath with less activity,
- rapid weight gain (five pounds per week or three pounds overnight),
- needing an increasing number of pillows to sleep at night,
- waking at night gasping for air, or
- swollen legs or feet or bloating of the stomach.

Other symptoms, such as fever, chills, and cough with yellow or green sputum, may not be heart related but still warrant a call to the doctor's office.

If the person has shortness of breath at rest that has worsened over minutes to hours, call 911. If the shortness of breath is accompanied by ongoing lightheadedness or dizziness or a fainting spell, call 911.

Most cardiologists' offices have a nurse who works closely with the doctor and will listen to your concerns, ask questions, and call you back with the doctor's recommendations. In some cases, people with heart failure are assigned to a heart failure physician in addition to their cardiologist. In such cases, it is prudent to contact the heart failure physician and nurse about these concerns. They are best suited to help you manage these symptoms on a day-to-day basis.

When you call the doctor's office, be ready to provide the following information:

- name,
- date of birth,
- name of the person's primary cardiologist,
- name of the person's heart failure doctor, and
- name of the nurse you generally talk with about these matters.

You can further help the doctor and the rest of the health care team by answering these questions:

- How is the shortness of breath compared with the past?
- Is there swelling of the legs? Decreased appetite? Swelling of the abdomen? Nausea? Are these symptoms worse than before?
- What medicines does the person take regularly? Does the person take any medicines on an as-needed basis? Has he or she taken them recently? Any recent changes in medicines? Any new supplements? Any new over-the-counter medicines?
- Has the person had bypass surgery? Stents? A pacemaker or defibrillator?
- What is the person's current weight? What is his or her usual weight?
- What is the person's blood pressure at home? Heart rate?
- Has the person had a recent stress test? Echocardiogram? Cardiac catheterization?
- Has the person had recent blood work? Who did it? Do you have the results with you?
- Has the person been hospitalized in the past for similar symptoms? If so, what was done at that time?
- Any recent changes to the person's diet?
- Does a home health nurse work with the person?

What Treatment Plan Will the Doctor Likely Create?

You may be advised to take one or more of these steps:

- Take the person to see the doctor, nurse practitioner, or physician assistant.

- Have the person admitted to the hospital.
- Increase dosages of current medicines or add new ones such as furosemide (Lasix), bumetanide (Bumex), toresemide (Demadex), or metolazone (Zaroxolyn).
- Improve blood pressure control by increasing dosages of current medicines or adding new ones.
- Take the person to have a chest X-ray, EKG (electrocardiogram), or echocardiogram.
- Take the person to have blood tests such as a basic metabolic panel or a blood test to measure B-type natriuretic peptide.

How Can I Help the Person in This Situation?

You have a major role in recognizing the person's changing symptoms. You are the eyes and ears of the health care team at home and a link between the health care system and the person's home.

You can look out for triggers for shortness of breath, such as a change in medicines or diet, increased alcohol intake, running out of medicines, and tobacco use. You can gather information, contact the doctor's office, and anticipate possible solutions that the doctor may suggest and help the person implement them.

If the doctor suggests a cause for this instance of dyspnea, you can help the person avoid it in the future (e.g., if a medicine change caused this episode, you can ensure that other members of the health care team do not mistakenly prescribe that medicine).

You can help the person with day-to-day activities while he recovers from the dyspnea. You may also track the impact of a treatment on symptoms and report it to the doctor's office as needed. As the person recovers, you can begin letting the person take over self-care and increase their daily activities.

PALPITATIONS

A palpitation is a sensation of abnormal heartbeats. People may say that their heart is beating too hard or fast, pounding, fluttering, skipping, flip-flopping, jumping out of their chest, or fluttering in their neck or throat.

Palpitations indicate an abnormal (regular or irregular) heart rhythm and may cause shortness of breath, chest pain, lightheadedness, or dizziness. In rare cases, people may pass out.

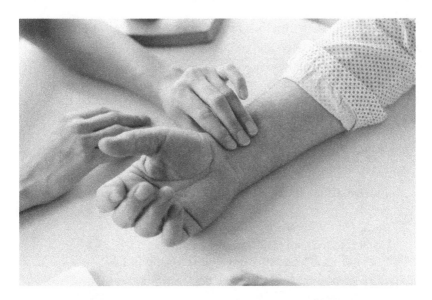

Figure 2.1. If possible, when someone is experiencing palpitations, check the person's pulse. © *iStock/Getty Images Plus/foremniakowski*

How Do Heart Problems Cause Palpitations?

Palpitations are caused by an abnormal heart rhythm that can arise from the upper or lower chambers of the heart. Depending on the type of abnormal rhythm, palpitations may be due to an abnormal heart circuit from birth but in some cases are caused by conditions such as a leaky valve, weak pumping of the heart, or sleep apnea.

Palpitations can also be caused by:

- anxiety, stress, and panic attacks;
- caffeine, alcohol, and medicines such as amphetamines;
- thyroid problems;
- fever;
- dehydration;
- vigorous exercise;
- pregnancy;
- anemia;
- medicines containing amphetamine (e.g., diet pills, decongestants); or
- certain herbal supplements.

What Kind of Heart Rhythm Problems Cause Palpitations? Should I Worry?

When the palpitation is described as a skipped beat, it may be from an extra beat coming from the upper (premature atrial contraction) or lower chamber (premature ventricular contraction) of the heart. This sensation lasts for a second or so, is generally benign, and only rarely requires treatment.

Palpitations described as ongoing, continuous, fluttering sensations of the heart may arise from rapid heartbeats coming from the upper or lower chamber of the heart. They include:

- **Supraventricular Tachycardia**
  - Regular rhythm coming from the upper chambers
  - Caused by an abnormal circuit in the heart
  - Can be treated with medicine or ablation
  - Does not affect longevity but may affect quality of life

- **Atrial Fibrillation**
  - Irregular rhythm coming from the upper chamber of the heart
  - Can be caused by factors such as a leaky heart valve, sleep apnea, or recent surgery
  - Can be associated with stroke and require blood thinners to prevent stroke
  - May affect quality of life
  - Can be treated with medicine or ablation

- **Atrial Flutter**
  - Regular rhythm coming from the upper chamber of the heart
  - Can be associated with stroke and require blood thinners to prevent stroke
  - May affect quality of life
  - Can be treated with medicine or ablation

- **Ventricular Tachycardia**
  - Rare but more likely in those with heart failure or prior heart attack
  - Regular rhythm coming from the lower chamber of the heart
  - Can be life threatening in people with previous heart attack or an otherwise weak heart
  - May affect longevity and quality of life in those with other heart conditions
  - Can be treated with medicine or ablation
  - If the person has had a heart attack or weak pumping of the heart, the doctor will recommend a defibrillator.

When Should I Call for Help?

If the person:

- Has passed out or feels like he is going to, call 911.
- Has ongoing palpitations with extreme shortness of breath or chest pain, call 911.
- Gets more than one shock from the implanted defibrillator, call 911.
- Feels lightheaded, call the doctor's office.
- Gets shocked from the implanted defibrillator and the palpitations have resolved, call the doctor's office.

When you call the doctor's office, be ready to answer the following questions:

- What is the person's name?
- What is the person's date of birth?
- Who is the person's primary cardiologist?
- Who is the person's heart failure doctor?
- Who is the nurse you generally talk with about these matters?
- Has the person had bypass surgery? Stents?
- Does the person have a pacemaker, defibrillator, or implanted monitor? If so, who assesses the device?

When you go to the emergency department or doctor's office, be prepared to answer the following questions:

- Did the person have chest pain, pressure, and shortness of breath with the palpitations?
- Did the person feel lightheaded or dizzy or pass out or feel like he was going to pass out during the palpitations?
- Did the palpitations start suddenly or gradually? Did they stop suddenly or gradually? How long did the episodes last?
- Is this the first time this has happened? How often do these episodes occur?
- What medicines does the person take regularly? Does he take any medicines on an as-needed basis? Has he taken them recently? Any recent changes in medicines? Has he used any natural supplements or over-the-counter medicines recently?

- Has the person had twenty-four- or forty-eight-hour Holter monitoring in the past for similar symptoms? Has the person had a fourteen- or twenty-eight-day event monitor in the past for similar symptoms?
- Has the person had ablations in the past for similar symptoms?

What Treatments Will the Doctor Recommend?

You will likely be asked to take the person to the doctor's office for an in-person examination, where the doctor may ask the questions listed previously in the chapter.

In addition, if the person has a pacemaker, defibrillator, or monitor, the doctor will check it or ask someone to check it. She may recommend a blood test to look for anemia or problems with the thyroid or electrolytes. She may prescribe other tests (e.g., electrocardiogram, echocardiogram, cardiac catheterization) and may recommend more specific tests related to palpitations such as:

- **Holter monitor:** The person will wear this for twenty-four or forty-eight hours and track when he feels palpitations. This is a good test if the person has several episodes a day. See chapter 5 on Holter monitoring for details.
- **Event recording:** The person will wear this monitor for two or four weeks and make recordings when he feels palpitations. The doctor will try to correlate the symptoms with any heart rhythm problems. This is a good test if the person has episodes once a week or so and is able to push a button on the machine to make a recording when he has symptoms.
- **Implantable loop recorder:** This surgically implanted monitor will remain in place under the skin for three years or until the correlation between the palpitations and an abnormal heart rhythm is made.

How Can I Help the Person in This Situation?

During palpitations, you can observe whether the person is dizzy, incoherent, short of breath, or close to passing out or whether he has passed out. In such cases, you should call 911.

If no such symptoms are present, you can help the person relax, which may stop the palpitations. If the episodes do not stop, have the person lie down and relax to prevent stress and anxiety related to the episode. If the doctor has prescribed a medicine to be used during episodes, you should give it to the person. If the episode does not stop, you may call the doctor's office or take the person to the emergency department.

If the episode stops on its own, you can record the details of the event (e.g., any chest pain or pressure, shortness of breath, dizziness) for the doctor. You should also note whether the onset was sudden or gradual and whether it stopped on its own.

It is important to note the duration of the episode and how often episodes occur. Further, if a monitor is prescribed, you should understand how to use it and ensure that the person uses it appropriately. If the doctor says that the palpitations are not concerning, you should remind the person of this and calm him during the next episode.

LEG SWELLING

Swelling of the feet, called pedal edema, can be a sign of fluid buildup in people with heart disease. It may affect one or both feet and go up into the legs. People feel heaviness in the legs and may complain of clothes feeling tight or socks leaving a dent. If leg swelling affects the ankle or knee joints, people may find movement difficult. Some people experience abdominal swelling or bloating instead of leg swelling.

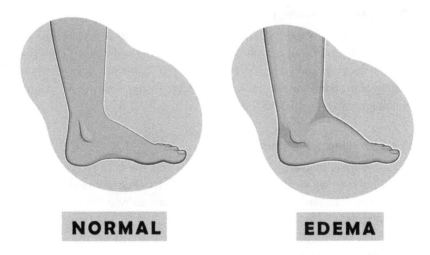

Figure 2.2. Swelling of the feet, called pedal edema, can be a sign of fluid buildup in people with heart disease. © *iStock/Getty Images Plus/ Chorna Olena*

Leg swelling can occur in people with heart conditions such as:

- heart failure,
- leaky heart valves, and
- pericarditis (inflammation of the sac around the heart).

However, leg swelling can also be caused by:

- kidney problems,
- liver problems,
- lung problems,
- low thyroid levels,
- pregnancy,
- being overweight,
- medicines such as steroids or painkillers (e.g., ibuprofen), or
- vein problems.

Other conditions that may cause leg swelling include:

- standing or sitting for long periods,
- inactivity, and
- inflammation in the leg tissues due to orthopedic problems (e.g., torn anterior cruciate ligament, gout).

Why Does Leg Swelling Occur?

When the heart is weak, it cannot pump enough blood to the kidneys. In turn, the kidneys cannot get rid of the fluid from the body. This fluid is retained in the body and causes swelling in the legs. Some people may notice swelling of the hands or abdomen first. Caregivers may notice rapid weight gain, fatigue, and shortness of breath.

Is Leg Swelling a Problem?

Yes, leg swelling indicates underlying disease and needs to be taken seriously. Moreover, leg swelling can increase the risk of falling due to a loss of balance and decreased sensation in the feet. Occasionally, it causes ulcers in the lower legs.

When Should I Contact the Doctor's Office?

Leg swelling is not an emergency when it happens gradually. However, when it occurs in one leg and progresses rapidly, it can be concerning. If leg swelling occurs along with chest pain, shortness of breath, dizziness, or coughing up blood, it may indicate a clot in the lungs and needs to be addressed immediately.

People with a previous heart condition should contact the doctor's office when they notice leg swelling.

When you call the doctor's office, be prepared to answer the following questions:

- What is the person's name?
- What is the person's date of birth?
- Who is the person's primary cardiologist?
- Who is the nurse you generally talk with about these matters?
- Has the person had bypass surgery? Stents?
- Does the person have chest pain, pressure, dizziness, shortness of breath, or cough?
- Are both legs affected?
- Did the leg swelling start suddenly or gradually?
- What does the person weigh? What is his usual weight?
- What medicines does the person take regularly? Does he take any water pills (diuretics) on an as-needed basis? Has he taken them recently? Any recent changes in medicines? Any increase in the use of painkillers? Has he used any natural supplements or over-the-counter medicines recently?
- Does he have kidney or liver problems?

What Treatment Is Recommended for Leg Swelling?

The doctor may recommend that the person undergo ultrasound of the legs to look for blood clots and blood tests to check kidney, liver, and thyroid function. Red blood cell and protein levels in the blood may be checked. People with leg swelling for the first time may be asked to have an echocardiogram to look for leaky valves and assess the pumping function of the heart.

To reduce leg swelling, the person may be asked to:

- consume less salt (see chapter 6 on diet for more information);
- elevate the legs at night by keeping a pillow under them when lying down;
- wear graded elastic compression stockings, which are tighter in the lower legs than in the thighs;
- avoid standing for prolonged periods;

- increase their activity level;
- change use of painkillers; or
- take an increased dose of diuretics.

PASSING OUT

Syncope is the medical term for sudden loss of consciousness, passing out, blacking out, or fainting. The episode may come out of nowhere for some people. However, many people are cold and clammy or feel lightheaded and dizzy before they faint. Others may have these symptoms before they pass out:

- a sense of warmth all over the body,
- blurred vision,
- fluttering of the heart or rapid heartbeat,
- nausea or vomiting, or
- tunnel vision, like everything is going dark around them.

Bystanders may notice that the person's face turns pale or blue during the episode. Jerky movements, as if the person is having a seizure after they faint, may be observed. It is important to note if the person lost control of their bowels or bladder after he passed out. When people regain consciousness, they may feel exhausted, while others can return to normal after the initial confusion has worn off.

The underlying reason for loss of consciousness is low blood flow to the brain. This decrease in blood flow may be caused by a low heart rate or low blood pressure.

A low heart rate may be due to:

- an abnormality in the heart's electrical system,
- medicines used to treat high blood pressure and/or a heart condition,
- an interaction between different medicines,
- electrolyte abnormalities,
- low thyroid levels (rare), or
- Lyme disease (very rare).

Low blood pressure may be due to:

- dehydration from excessive heat exposure or low fluid intake,
- use of excessive amounts of diuretics,

- medicines for high blood pressure and/or a heart condition,
- an interaction between medicines, including over-the-counter varieties, or
- a sudden change in position from sitting or lying down to standing up.

A combination of low heart rate and blood pressure may be due to:

- an overactive nervous system triggered by seeing blood, having blood drawn, pain, fear, or sudden emotional stress;
- prolonged standing;
- straining during a bowel movement;
- urination;
- nausea and vomiting;
- neurologic causes; or
- unidentified causes.

How Can Syncope Be Prevented?

The person may be able to avoid some instances of syncope by lying down and raising his legs when he starts feeling dizzy or sitting down and putting his head between his knees. If he feels fluttering in the chest or a rapid heartbeat, sitting down may help him avoid fainting.

When Is the Fainting Spell Worrisome Enough to Call for Help?

Call 911 if:

- It is the first episode of syncope.
- The person has a known heart condition.
- The person is injured from fainting and falling.

If the person with syncope has a defibrillator and it fires, call the doctor's office immediately. If a person with known vasovagal syncope has another episode of syncope, you may not need to call the doctor's office immediately.

When you call the doctor's office to report syncope, be ready to answer these questions:

- What is the person's name?
- What is the person's date of birth?
- Who is the person's primary cardiologist?

- Who is the person's electrophysiologist, if any?
- Who is the nurse you generally talk with about these matters?
- Has the person had bypass surgery? Stents?
- Does the person have a pacemaker, defibrillator, or implanted monitor? If so, do you have a card from the device company? Also, who generally checks this device?

In cases of syncope, the more information you can offer the doctor, the better the diagnosis.

When you go to the emergency department or doctor's office, be prepared to answer the following questions:

- Did the person feel unwell over the past twenty-four hours? Did the person have nausea or vomiting before or after the fainting spell? Lightheaded or dizzy? Tunnel vision or blurry vision? Loss of bowel or bladder control, palpitations, chest pain, pressure, or shortness of breath with the episode?
- Did the person fall? Was he injured?
- Is this the first instance of fainting? If not, how often does it happen? Was the person examined and treated afterward? What was the reason for fainting in the past?
- What medicines does the person take regularly, either on an as-needed basis or over the counter? Any recent changes in medicines?

What Kind of Treatments Will the Doctor Likely Recommend?

You may be asked to bring the person to the doctor's office for an examination, where the doctor may ask the previously mentioned questions. The more detailed the answers, the better. If the person has a pacemaker, defibrillator, or monitor, the doctor will check it. She may recommend hospitalization or evaluate the person in the clinic.

The following tests may be conducted:

- blood tests to look for anemia, dehydration, or thyroid problems;
- an electrocardiogram to check the heart's rate and rhythm;
- an echocardiogram, an ultrasound test discussed in chapter 5 that checks heart pumping and for previous heart attacks and valve problems; or
- an exercise stress test to look for blockages in the coronary arteries and any abnormal heart rhythms with exercise.

The following tests may also be performed to uncover the cause of syncope:

- **Holter monitoring:** The person wears this monitor for twenty-four or forty-eight hours, noting when he feels lightheaded or dizzy. The doctor tries to correlate the symptoms with any heart rhythm problems. This is a good test if the person has episodes more than once a day. See chapter 5 on Holter monitoring for details.
- **Event recording:** The person wears a monitor for two or four weeks, making recordings when he feels lightheaded or dizzy. This is a good test if the person has episodes once a week or so.
- **Implantable loop recorder:** This surgically implanted monitor remains under the skin for three years or until the correlation between the syncope and abnormal heart rhythm is discovered.
- **Electrophysiology study:** In people with a known heart condition, syncope is worrisome. More intensive workup, including an invasive electrophysiology study, may be done. Here, the doctor places catheters inside the heart via small tubes in the right or left leg. She tries to cause abnormal heart rhythms through this study, which may help uncover the cause of syncope.

What Treatment Options Will Be Offered?

Depending on the cause of syncope, these treatments may be offered:

Condition	Treatment Options
Dehydration	Change of medicines, increased fluid intake, compression stockings
Low blood pressure	Change of medicines or their dosages
Vasovagal syncope	Increased fluid intake, compression stockings, foot exercises before standing, new medicines, avoidance of triggers
Low heart rate	Change of medicine, pacemaker insertion
Anemia	Blood transfusion, iron supplementation, other medications
Rapid heartbeat	Ablation, defibrillator insertion

How Can I Help in This Situation?

In syncope more than in any other condition, you function as the eyes and ears of the health care team. You can observe whether the person was nauseous, dizzy, incoherent, short of breath, having chest pain, or looking pale before fainting.

You can verify whether the person actually lost consciousness or just came close to it. In such cases, you should call 911. You can report whether the person had seizure-like movements or bowel or bladder incontinence during syncope. You should ensure that the person is laid flat and does not try to stand up right away.

If you are trained, you can measure heart rate and blood pressure once the person has regained consciousness. If appropriate, you should bring the person to the emergency department or call 911.

In the emergency department, you can offer the previously mentioned details to the doctors involved in the person's care. Further, if a monitor is prescribed, you should understand how to use it and ensure that the person uses it appropriately. If a trigger is identified for the syncope, you can help the person avoid it in the future. If the doctor says that the episode is not concerning, you should remind the person of this and calm him if another episode occurs.

Three

TAKING CARE OF YOURSELF

I was completely focused on him, and then I felt irritated and frustrated by him. We fought often. Now that I take breaks, things are much better. I think that caregivers need to take breaks and do some things for themselves away from the person.

—*Mary, wife of a person with advanced heart disease*

Being a caregiver is an immense responsibility and involves tremendous sacrifices. It is a commitment of time and energy for a long, unknown duration. As a caregiver, you have to think about your responsibility as a marathon rather than a sprint.

The best care is provided not by selfless and self-sacrificial caregivers but by those who strike a balance between self-care and care of the person. Maintaining balance and seeking support from others can help you maintain good physical and emotional health while caring for the person. It will make you an effective caregiver for years to come. Follow the tips in this chapter to help you get on the right path early and prevent burnout.

CARING FOR YOUR OWN PHYSICAL HEALTH

One of the biggest problems in caregiving is becoming sick yourself. It is important to be vigilant against this risk. While caring for your loved one, keep your own needs in mind. Recognize when you are hungry, thirsty, or tired. Take a break to care for your body. There will be times when you will be tired and need a longer break. Acknowledge this, and ask for help.

Exercise is good for the body and mind. It relieves stress and boosts energy levels. Caregivers who exercise are more optimistic and have a more positive outlook toward the person's disease. Even a brisk walk in the neighborhood for thirty minutes will yield positive results.

Get seven or eight hours of sleep each night. It will act as a buffer against stress and burnout.

Eat a Healthy Diet

A heart-healthy diet, such as the one described in chapter 6, is not only a part of the treatment for heart disease but also helps prevent heart disease. If you share meals with the person, adopt the heart-healthy diet for benefits for the person as well as you. Here are some tips:

- While managing multiple tasks, it is easy to get into the habit of eating fast food, which is unhealthy. Leave the junk food in the grocery store, and buy only nutritious food, including an adequate supply of fruits and vegetables.
- Make a meal plan for the week. Keep healthy recipes handy when you plan and take a list of needed foods to the grocery store. Choose whole-grain ingredients like whole-wheat flour, oatmeal, and whole cornmeal for making baked goods such as bread and muffins. Use healthy fats like olive oil rather than saturated fats, and avoid processed foods.
- Cook in large batches and freeze meals for a few days so you do not have to resort to junk food under time pressure.
- Keep nutritious snacks (e.g., ready-to-eat chopped fruits and vegetables, unsalted nuts) on hand to eat on the go, if needed. A banana, frozen berries, and low-fat yogurt can make a healthy and refreshing smoothie in minutes.

Following these simple tips and the guidelines in chapter 6, you will be able to cook healthy meals for yourself and your loved ones. You will be able to keep your loved one on track with their dietary requirements while maintaining a healthy weight and energy level yourself.

CARING FOR YOUR OWN MENTAL HEALTH

It is easy to become overwhelmed by the responsibilities of caregiving. Plan for the future, but live in the moment. The future may seem overwhelming, so it is important to take one day at a time. Maintaining a positive attitude is critical to effectively manage the responsibilities of caregiving day after day, week after week.

Recognize that heart disease is a chronic condition with ups and downs. There is no "same old, same old" in heart disease. You have to cope with daily changes, encouraging self-management one day and stepping in to take control on another. Caregivers who go with the flow and embrace the daily variations of heart disease experience less frustration and cope better.

Adjusting to your role and learning how to navigate the disease and the health care system takes time. Throughout this process, remember that you are doing the best you can. Remember that you have empowered yourself with knowledge about heart disease, that you know what needs to be done to help your loved one, and that you have support all around you.

Caregivers show a range of reactions to their role. On some days, you may feel stoic, while on other days, you may feel angry, frustrated, lonely, and burdened. Know that all caregivers go through these emotions. Take one day at a time, and talk with friends and family or other caregivers in your situation.

The person's health care team has resources to help you get support from local agencies when you need it. Both formal and informal support systems will help you cope.

With the stress and anxiety over the health of the person, it is easy to get depressed. Watch for these signs of depression in yourself:

- sleeping too much or having insomnia;
- feeling tired and worn out all the time;
- irritability;
- restlessness;
- feelings of guilt;
- hopelessness;
- avoidance of activities once found enjoyable;
- use of medicines or alcohol;
- no appetite or eating too much, leading to excessive weight loss or gain; or
- thoughts of ending your life.

If you have these thoughts, seek help from a professional counselor, psychotherapist, or psychiatrist.

Do Not Put Your Own Life on Hold

By getting completely absorbed in the task of caregiving to the exclusion of all else, caregivers feel that they have put their own life on hold. This may lead to frustration over the disease and even the loved one. To avoid such negative emotions, keep the essentials of your life going. Keep your doctor's appointments, manage your finances, and keep up with your friends, even when (and especially when) you feel overwhelmed with caregiving responsibilities. Set personal goals, however small, and work toward them. This will guard against caregiver burnout and give you a sense of accomplishment.

Make Time for Yourself

Caregivers need to recognize the importance of caring for themselves so they can better care for the person. In the early stages of the disease, the person can manage to prepare simple meals, go to the bathroom, and do light work.

You should recognize good days when the person is doing well and has no alarming symptoms. Encourage the person to do these activities so you can make some time for yourself.

Later in the disease, when your loved one needs more help, taking some personal time can be therapeutic. Even if it is for just a few minutes a day, do what you find relaxing or cathartic. This can come in the form of small pleasures such as reading a favorite magazine, going for a short walk, swimming, or relaxing in a hot tub. Music, gardening, games, puzzles, coloring, painting, and crafts are some activities that may rejuvenate you.

Do not feel guilty about taking time away from your loved one. Caregivers who do not make time for themselves react negatively to the situation and loved one. They experience fatigue and frustration, which in turn affects their ability to care for the patient as well as their relationship with the patient. Conversely, caregivers who take time for self-care provide better care and enjoy their life.

Get Outside and Connect with the World

It is easy to stay inside taking care of your loved one day after day. After a while, it even comes naturally, and there is a tendency to put off everything else. However, it is critical to get out and connect with others. It may be as simple as meeting a friend for a cup of coffee, watching a movie, going birthday card shopping, or attending church activities.

Social ties will help you in difficult times and provide a much-needed break from caregiving responsibilities.

ORGANIZATION TIPS

Caregiving is an additional task to all the other to-dos of life. It can be rewarding but may cause stress and strife in day-to-day life. It can also bring a feeling of loss of control over time and life. Most caregivers find that staying organized can reestablish this sense of control, reduce stress, and help accomplish caregiving, self-care, and other activities of life. The small up-front work of staying organized can prevent last-minute emergencies. Here are some of the ways caregivers have stayed organized.

Time

An up-to-date, well-maintained calendar decreases the possibility of missing appointments and the need to be at two places at once. Multiple calendars for different aspects of your life (e.g., work, kids, caregiving) may result in unforeseen conflicts. Create one calendar for all your activities. Despite the obvious appeal of paper calendars, electronic calendars have a lot of advantages. Electronic calendars can be updated on the go and shared with other family members who participate in caregiving duties. Some electronic calendars also take input from your e-mail and automatically populate the event. Google and Outlook Calendar are freely available shareable electronic calendars. Specific caregiving apps such as Carezone can help manage your calendar, medication list, test results, insurance information, and emergency contacts. The Lotsa app from Lotsa Helping Hands can coordinate efforts when there are multiple caregivers. A printed copy of the calendar in a prominent place can be a visual aid to remind you of the tasks of the days, weeks, and months ahead and help relieve the stress of remembering events and tasks.

Information

As a caregiver, you are likely to be responsible for providing all the information about your loved one's health to health care providers. The electronic medical records at doctors' offices are unlikely to be shared between doctors and, hence, an updated lab test or medication list from one clinic does not reach the other. Unfortunately, you are likely to be the only accurate source of up-to-date information. Keeping medical information organized can be challenging, but there are ways to make it manageable. For caregivers who are digital-minded, Get Real Health (getrealhealth.com/instantphr) and FollowMyHealth (followmyhealth.com) can be a repository of all health information that can be easily shared.

Other caregivers have found it useful to use an accordion folder or three-ring binder with sections such as these:

- Medicines: Use the template at the end of this section to keep an updated list of medicines. Update this list every time a doctor changes a dose or adds or stops a medicine. Review the list with what the patient is taking on a monthly basis.
- Allergies: Allergies to medicines, food, or materials (e.g., latex, adhesives) should be noted.

- Doctors: Use the template at the end of this section to keep lists and contact information of all health care providers caring for your loved one.
- Medical history: Use the template at the end of this section to keep a list of the person's medical history, including previous surgeries.
- Recent lab tests: Keep the results of basic blood tests (blood count, kidney function, blood electrolytes), radiology results (radiographs, computed tomographic [CT] blood scans, magnetic resonance imaging), cardiac tests (echocardiograms, stress tests, coronary angiograms, coronary artery bypass grafting reports), and hospital release summaries.
- Legal information: Keep the following forms filed: DNR order, POLST form, and medical power of attorney document.
- Insurance-related information: Keep copies of current insurance cards and prescription plan cards.
- Photo identification card: This document is generally required when checking in to the doctor's office and emergency department. Keep a copy of the person's driver's license or any state-issued photo identification card handy.

With the amount of information coming your way, it is very easy to lose track of all the data quickly. Some caregivers find that carrying a notebook and pen and taking notes relieves them of the burden of remembering everything. Buy a small notebook that can be easily placed in a pocket or purse. Some caregivers take notes on their phone so they do not have to remember to carry the notebook and pen.

Lists

In the busy life of a caregiver, it is impossible to thrive without making lists. Tech-savvy caregivers use one of the many apps available to help with this task (e.g., Todoist, Tick, Microsoft To Do, Any.do). Some apps synchronize with the digital calendar. Other caregivers keep paper lists for common tasks (e.g., groceries and medicines to pick up, questions to ask health care providers). Some caregivers may find it worthwhile to learn an app because it relieves them of the burden of carrying or remembering to populate the lists. Such an electronic list that is portable and difficult to lose has obvious advantages.

Organizing Medicines

The caregiver should work with the patient to track medicine use. With guidance from health care providers and pharmacists, the caregiver should understand how medicines must be taken and routinely help the patient set up the pillbox for the next week. Use daily reminders with an alarm clock or preferably an app on the phone to take the medicines on time. The caregiver should ensure an ample supply of medicines. If any medicines are about to run out, order refills in a timely manner. Apps that help with tracking medicines (e.g., CareZone) may also offer notices when a refill needs to be requested. In some cases, pharmacies can help you synchronize the prescription refill times for multiple medicines so all prescriptions can be picked up once a month. Maintain a list of medicines, and update it whenever a change is made by any provider. Bring the updated list to each and every clinic visit.

Emergency Planning

In patients with heart disease, emergencies are not uncommon. Caregivers need to be prepared and plan accordingly. Some caregivers prefer to have an emergency bag ready at all times with a current copy of the patient file mentioned previously, complete with the patient's medical history, current medicine list, physician information, insurance-related documents, personal identification, legal documents, and pen and paper. Some caregivers suggest having cash, bottled water, healthy snacks, puzzles, or reading material ready in cases of long waits in the emergency department. A change of clothes for the person may also help. Keep the emergency kit where others (e.g., paramedics, other caregivers) can access it in your absence. Despite having these plans and getting organized, keep in mind that there will be unusual circumstances for which you may feel unprepared. At such times, recognize that this too is to be expected. Accept such detours, learn from them, and move on without judgment.

Procrastination is the beginning of a cascade to avoid. Small tasks accumulated through procrastination will overwhelm you. Keep a notebook documenting preferences, habits, and proclivities of your loved one for daily activities. Such information can be helpful to other caregivers at home or in the hospital. Create a backup plan in case you are not available. Look for friends and neighbors who can help if needed. Keep a list with their contact information on hand. Anticipate future needs for the patient and plan accordingly. (For example, is surgery in the future? If so, read about it in this book and anticipate the patient's needs before and after surgery and change your schedule accordingly.)

Information Templates

MEDICINE RECORD

Medicine	Dose	Date started	Reason for taking	Side effects/ notes
Metoprolol	25 mg twice a day	12/12/2012	Heart disease	

DOCTORS AND OTHER HEALTH CARE PROVIDERS

Primary care physician	Dr. Johnson	xxx-xxx-xxxx
Cardiologist	Dr. Smith	xxx-xxx-xxxx
Pharmacy	Greenmart	xxx-xxx-xxxx
Home care agency		

MEDICAL HISTORY

Disease	Since	Medicine	Notes
Diabetes	2004	Insulin, metformin	Dr. Smith

SURGICAL HISTORY

Surgery	Date	Surgeon	Notes
Bypass	2010	Dr. Johnson	Three vessels, aortic valve replaced
Angioplasty	2006	Dr. Kumar	Stent placed

ASKING FOR HELP

Caregiving is a tough job with physical, emotional, and financial effects. Two-thirds of caregivers suffer from increased stress, and half of them skip their own doctors' appointments. Furthermore, about two-thirds of caregivers have financial worries due to caregiving. All of this can lead to burnout.

Many resources are available to provide emotional and social support as well as much needed respite from caregiving. Being aware of local and statewide support systems and services can help you feel equipped for your pivotal role.

Starting Points

The person's health care provider is a good place to start in finding resources. In addition, every county or region in the country has organizations that can provide guidance (e.g., American Heart Association). Support groups in most communities help caregivers talk with others having similar experiences. Multiple resources are available online as well as in the community. A list of organizations, associations, and agencies at the end of this section will help you locate these services.

Family, Friends, and Other Resources

It is important to identify friends and family who not only offer emotional support but also help with tasks involved in caregiving. Engaging them early will ease your burden and make it easy to ask for help when needed. Engaging others will also allow your loved one to continue to have other connections in life. Some caregivers have found it useful to make a list of the tasks to be performed every week and share it with others on the team to seek help in accomplishing them. Create an online help calendar to coordinate everyone's tasks throughout the week.

Consider using adult daycare services in your area to allow you to take care of your own needs. Your health care team, especially a social worker, can help you find an appropriate center. You can also visit nadsa.org/locator/ to locate adult daycare. Occasionally, take a weekend to do something for yourself. Your support team of friends and family can care for your loved one during your break. Alternatively, you can seek respite care. A volunteer program from Senior Corps offers respite care with volunteer seniors. The caregiver may find more information about this program at nationalservice.gov/

programs/senior-corps. The National Family Caregiver Support Program (acl.gov/programs/support-caregivers/national-family-caregiver-support -program) provides federal funds to each state to support a caregiver respite care program with trained professionals. Contact your local Area Agency on Aging to enroll.

In addition, some community-based groups provide respite care via screened and trained volunteers. If your loved one requires more intense medical care, the Visiting Nurses Association of America (vnaa.org/) and its affiliates can help. The patient's health care team can be a great resource for finding groups in your area. The ARCH Respite Network (archrespite.org/) can help you find respite care providers and ways to pay for it.

It is important to recognize that there are other caregivers who have been down this path and learned from it. It is important to seek support and learn from their experiences. Support groups are available online and in communities.

- The American Heart Association maintains a message board on which caregivers can exchange ideas and find support at supportnetwork.heart. org/connect-with-people-like-me/caregiver/caregiver-heart/.
- Mended Hearts is a person advocacy group that offers online support, lectures, and conferences in local communities. Find more information at mendedhearts.org/.
- The Caregiver Action Network is a family caregiver organization, helping caregivers nationwide care for people with different diseases and disabilities. A nonprofit organization, it provides education, peer support, and resources. Find more information at caregiveraction.org/resources.

Help at Work

About twenty-four million Americans are caring for a loved one while also trying to earn a living. The onerous work of caregiving leads to lower productivity at work due to the emotional burden and physical exhaustion of caregiving. It is important to seek alternative work arrangements to balance your productivity at work with caregiving at home. Many workplaces have options to help you achieve this goal. Consider discussing these options with your supervisor or human resources representative.

Flexible Work Hours

Consider a compressed workweek (e.g., four ten-hour days or three twelve-hour days). Some caregivers alter their office hours to come in early, leave in the early afternoon, and have time for caregiving. Alternatively, some jobs allow working from home (telecommuting).

Counseling Services

Many workplaces have an employee assistance program or other resources for caregivers at no extra cost. A well-run employee assistance program can help reduce stress, recognize depression, and better manage time. If your workplace offers a support group for caregivers, you can benefit from the experience of others in similar situations. If there isn't one, consider starting one.

Using Paid Time Off for Caregiving

Caregivers may be allowed to use paid sick days or vacation leave to care for a loved one. In some states, employees can take paid time off through the family leave insurance program. The number of states offering such benefits is expanding (aarp.org/caregiving/financial-legal/info-2019/paid-family-leave-laws.html). Alternatively, you can explore taking unpaid leave under the federally mandated Family and Medical Leave Act (FMLA). This federal law entitles workers to take unpaid leave of as long as twelve weeks per year to care for their loved ones with serious health conditions. Unfortunately, FMLA does not cover leave taken to care for in-laws. The law protects workers from losing their job or health benefits during this time. Visit the employee guide to FMLA at dol.gov/sites/dolgov/files/WHD/legacy/files/employeeguide.pdf for more information.

Alternative Ideas

Employers may be able to use ideas and tool kits from AARP to support employee caregivers at home (aarp.org/caregiving/life-balance/info-2017/ways-to-support-working-caregivers-lh.html).

Useful Websites and Resources

- The American Heart Association maintains a message board on which caregivers can exchange ideas and find support at supportnetwork.heart.org/connect-with-people-like-me/caregiver/caregiver-heart/.
- Mended Hearts is a patient advocacy group that offers online support, lectures, and conferences in local communities. Find more information at mendedhearts.org/.

- The Caregiver Action Network is a family caregiver organization supporting caregivers nationwide in caring for people with different diseases and disabilities. A nonprofit organization, it provides education, peer support, and resources. Find more information at caregiveraction.org/resources or call 855-227-3640.
- AARP's family caregiving site offers legal checklists, information on care options, and an online community of support for family caregivers. Call 877-333-5885 or visit aarp.org/caregiving/.
- Eldercare Locator helps find local respite care providers, insurance counseling, transportation, and other services for patients and caregivers. Call 800-677-1116 or visit communityresourcefinder.org/.
- The Family Caregiver Alliance provides information, education, and support groups for family caregivers, including a state-by-state list of services. Call 800-445-8106 or visit caregiver.org/.
- The National Institute on Aging offers information related to health and caregiving. Call 800-222-2225 or visit www.nia.nih.gov/.
- The Well Spouse Association offers social support to spouses acting as caregivers. Their online chatroom helps you connect with other spouses in a similar role. Call 800-838-0879 or visit wellspouse.org/.
- Medicare offers help locating quality home health agencies that provide patient care at home with certified nurses and aides. Visit medicare.gov/homehealthcompare/search.html.
- Medicaid can help people with limited income and assets pay for long-term care. The coverage may differ from state to state. Call your state Medicaid agency to see if you qualify. Find your state's Medicaid contact information at medicaid.gov/about-us/contact-us/contact-state-page.html.
- If the person is sixty-five or older, Medicare can help cover the cost of home health as well as skilled nursing services in some circumstances. Call 800-633-2273 to find out more.
- The National Academy of Elder Law Attorneys is a nonprofit association of lawyers and organizations that provides legal services (e.g., power of attorney, long-term care, other aging- and health-related issues). Visit www.naela.org/.
- The Administration on Aging provides an online clearinghouse for information on long-term care needs, financial coverage, and information on Medicare and Medicaid and multiple other issues. Visit longtermcare.acl.gov/ for more information.
- The National Center for Assisted Living, part of the American Health Care Association, offers many resources on finding assisted living

facilities, the cost of these facilities, and state programs. Visit ahcancal .org/ncal/Pages/index.aspx.

- A similar database is maintained at medicare.gov/nursinghomecompare /search.html to provide information about Medicare- and Medicaid-certified nursing homes around the country.
- The National Adult Day Services Association can help locate an adult daycare close to you. Visit https://www.nadsa.org/locator/.
- Senior Corps offers respite care with volunteer seniors. Visit nationalservice .gov/programs/senior-corps.
- The National Family Caregiver Support Program (acl.gov/programs/ support-caregivers/national-family-caregiver-support-program) provides federal funds to each state to support a caregiver respite care program with trained caregivers. Contact your local Area Agency on Aging to enroll.
- For more intense medical care at home, the Visiting Nurses Association of America (vnaa.org/) and its affiliates can help.
- The ARCH Respite Network (https://archrespite.org/) can help find respite care providers in your area and ways to pay for it.
- AARP offers a guide to help initiate conversations about life goals for patients, self-care for caregivers, and many other topics. Download the document at aarp.org/content/dam/aarp/home-and-family/caregiving /2012-10/PrepareToCare-Guide-FINAL.pdf to help prepare for your role as a caregiver.
- The Center to Advance Palliative Care offers a list of providers in your area who specialize in palliative care. Visit https://getpalliativecare.org/.
- Similarly, find quality Medicare-accepting hospice providers in your area at medicare.gov/hospiceCompare/.
- The Hospice Foundation of America provides a list of hospice providers and practical tips and advice for caregivers. Call 800-854-3402 or visit hospicefoundation.org/.

Four

SETTING GOALS

It was difficult to talk about it, but now I know what she wants. So when the time comes, we can follow her wishes. I think, as a caregiver, you have to figure out a way to have these conversations.

—*Michelle, whose aunt has advanced heart disease*

The disease course of a person with advanced heart disease includes many twists and turns; some are unexpected, while others are common.

GOALS OF CARE

For those with advanced heart disease, it is important to create goals so as to decrease futile care and needless suffering near the end-of-life. People often receive care at such times that physicians consider futile. This happens all too often because the goals at the end of life have been neither discussed nor documented. A person with heart disease should be encouraged to articulate their end-of-life wishes so that the caregiver can work with the health care providers to achieve those goals.

Some treatments help people with heart disease get better and prolong their lives. Some of these treatments, especially surgical ones, come with initial postoperative pain and discomfort and confinement to bed for a few days during recovery. If the person continues to enjoy good quality of life and wants to consider life-prolonging options, such curative treatment options would be appropriate. However, if the person has daily struggles that negatively affect quality of life and would rather focus on symptom relief and improved quality of life, such treatment options could be avoided. The goal of care needs to be defined to reflect this focus. Such articulated and documented goals should be the beacon guiding caregivers and family members in choosing among different types of treatment.

If there is no discussion or documentation of these goals, the family members and caregivers feel a great void and may choose options that are not in keeping with the person's goals and may lead to unnecessary suffering.

An individual's goals for end-of-life care vary depending on factors such as their value system, current quality of life, spirituality, previous experience with health care, and past interactions with others at the end of life. Sometimes, the person may voice a much simpler goal or preference in the form of spending time at home with family. The person and caregiver, along with the medical power of attorney, need to discuss end-of-life care and clearly understand these goals. Such conversations, though difficult, will avoid a more difficult and perplexing situation of guessing what the person would want when they can no longer voice their choices.

Experts have recommended starting such conversations with questions such as:

- What is most important to you now? What are your priorities?
- What are you most concerned about?
- Who knows your medical care preferences and can speak for you if you cannot speak for yourself?
- What level of medical intervention is desired when life is limited (e.g., would you want open-heart surgery)? Do you want to be fed with a tube? Do you want to be hooked up to a ventilator? Do you want dialysis? Do you want blood checks?
- If you are unconscious and have no chance of becoming conscious again, would you want further medical interventions?
- If medical treatments are becoming less beneficial (e.g., less than 50 percent), would you still want them?
- When would you want us to focus on symptom relief, comfort, and pain control?

WHAT IS ADVANCE CARE PLANNING?

It is critical to anticipate different future scenarios and the person's preferences in those situations. This process is called advance care planning. Here, the person discusses her care choices with her caregivers and health care proxies ahead of time. This helps them make choices based on those preferences when the person is not able to later on.

People may be reluctant to discuss these issues if they find them distressing. A caregiver should start the conversation after the initial diagnosis and facilitate review of the plans every six months or so.

In people with advanced heart disease, advance care planning involves shared decision-making among people, family members, health care proxies, and health care providers. The key steps are:

- recognizing the person's values, goals, and preferences;
- understanding scenarios the person may encounter;
- making specific plans based on the person's values, priorities, and preferences;
- documenting these plans in an advance directive or living will; and
- choosing a health care proxy who will make a decision if the person cannot.

Advance care planning should be done early in the course of heart disease treatment. People must recognize that these stated preferences can be changed over time. Making these choices early relieves caregivers and family members of making difficult choices in stressful circumstances.

People with advanced heart disease need to make decisions such as:

- What are the person's values and preferences regarding health care?
- What does she fear most about the future?
- Would anything be worse than death for her?

In case of cardiac arrest:

- Would she want to be revived with chest compressions and cardiopulmonary resuscitation (CPR)?
- Would she want a natural death?
- Would she want a tube placed down her throat to help her breathe?

If there is no hope for a meaningful recovery:

- Should all life-prolonging measures be continued?
- Should the team provide comfort measures only?
- Under what situations should the team switch to comfort measures only?
- Would she want another cardiac catheterization? A stent? Another open-heart surgery?
- Would she want a tracheostomy to be performed for long-term ventilation?
- Would she want a feeding tube?

- Would she want the ICD to shock her out of a fatal heart rhythm?
- If she has a left ventricular assist device, when would she want it turned off?
- What if she has a stroke?
- What if she has a life-threatening infection?
- Who is her health care proxy if she cannot speak for herself?

A nice tool for initiating this conversation with the person can be found at thelastvisit.com/wp-content/uploads/2014/09/5-Wishes-Advanced -Planning-Guide1.pdf.

The family is a critical part of these conversations. They can initiate these conversations and help the person make her choices.

POWER OF ATTORNEY, LIVING WILL, DNR AND DNI ORDERS, AND POLST

Different documents provide written, legally binding instructions for medical care when the person is unable to make those choices. Each one accomplishes a different task.

Power of Attorney

In this directive, the person names another person to make decisions for her when she cannot. This directive is also called a medical power of attorney, health care power of attorney, durable power of attorney, and health care proxy. The person nominated to make decisions may be called a health care agent, health care proxy, health care surrogate, or health care representative. Caregivers typically make the best power of attorney, but the person may choose someone else who is proactive about discussing difficult end-of-life issues and can be trusted to advocate for her when she cannot. The person may also choose one or more alternates in case the person with power of attorney cannot fulfill the role.

Living Will

A living will is a legally binding written document to declare the person's preferences for life-sustaining medical treatment. It spells out her preferences for organ and tissue donation and may address the use of CPR, mechanical ventilation, tube feeding, dialysis, antibiotics or antiviral medicines, comfort (palliative) care, hospice care, and donating her body for scientific study.

Do-Not-Resuscitate (DNR) and Do-Not-Intubate (DNI) Orders

These orders are generally part of a living will. However, if the person does not have a living will, she can tell her wishes to her doctor, and he can enter them as an order in her medical record. It is helpful to discuss this with the doctor every time she is hospitalized.

Physician Orders for Life-Sustaining Treatment (POLST)

The person may also request a physician to sign a POLST, an order about which measures should be taken by emergency or medical personnel, in keeping with her advance directive. This document should always be near the person (e.g., at home, next to her bed or on the refrigerator; at a nursing home, near her bed). It should be displayed prominently so it is easy for emergency personnel to find. A POLST may include the following:

- chest compressions and CPR,
- intubation and mechanical ventilation,
- transfer to an emergency department,
- admission to a hospital,
- tube feeding,
- use of antibiotics,
- pain management, and
- health care proxy name.

In emergencies, you can direct emergency medical personnel to provide care based on the POLST and living will.

HOW TO CREATE THESE DOCUMENTS

For advance directives, each state in the United States has a specific form. You do not need to hire a lawyer to create an advance directive. One can find the specific forms on websites such as these:

- aarp.org/caregiving/financial-legal/free-printable-advance-directives/ and
- caringinfo.org/i4a/pages/index.cfm?pageid=3289.

The caregiver or the person can print this form, discuss it with the health care proxy, and fill it out. Later, make an appointment with the doctor, and review the advance directive with the doctor to ensure that the completed form is in keeping with the person's preferences. Then give a copy to the doctor and health care proxy. The originals should be placed in an accessible location. The person should carry a copy when traveling; a wallet-sized card such as this one works well:

I Have an Advance Directive

Name: _____

Date of Birth:

Physician name: _____

Physician phone no.:

I have advance directives. Copies are held by:

Name: _____

Phone no: _____

My health care proxy is:

Name: _____

Phone no: _____

Figure 4.1. Patients should be encouraged to articulate their end-of-life wishes so that the caregiver can work with the health care providers to achieve those goals. *J Shah, MD*

Other wallet cards may be printed from theagelist.files.wordpress.com /2013/04/advance-directives-wallet-card.jpg. You can facilitate this process and ensure that the documents are in place.

Five

COMMON HEART CONDITIONS, TESTS, AND TREATMENTS

At first, it was overwhelming. The doctor tried to explain everything and the staff were explaining what to expect. But I just couldn't put it together. It was almost like they had a different language and I could not understand most of it. But after six months and multiple doctor visits, I got a hang of it. Now, I advise everyone to read up, so that they grasp what is being said and participate in making decisions.

—Nigel, whose grandfather has advanced heart disease

Having some knowledge of the various heart diseases and understanding the basics of the frequently used tests and treatments is important for the caregiver. It will help them grasp what the doctor is explaining and then ask the right questions. It will help the caregiver keep the person on track with following the doctor's recommendations. It will also help the caregiver be vigilant that the care is in keeping with the person's goals. In this chapter, we will discuss diseases that affect the heart muscle, valves, coronary artery, or electrical system of the heart. We will also discuss the pertinent cardiac tests and treatments commonly undertaken.

HEART FAILURE

Sometimes called congestive heart failure, this is an unfortunate term that may leave the person and caregivers despondent. However, understanding the condition will help you overcome the anxiety that these words provoke and navigate this disease with confidence. With appropriate care, a person with a diagnosis of heart failure can live a number of years with good quality of life.

Heart failure refers to a condition caused by the heart's inability to pump enough blood to satisfy the oxygen needs of the body. Hence, the body's organs do not get enough blood. The kidneys react by retaining water and salt in the body. This results in fluid building up in the legs and ankles, causing them to swell. Fluid builds up in the lungs and interferes with breathing, causing shortness of breath.

If untreated, heart failure causes the heart valves to leak and abnormal rhythm problems in the electrical system. Over time, other organs are damaged due to lack of oxygen.

The severity of heart failure is classified into one of four categories:

- **Class I:** Person has no symptoms and can carry out all activities without any problems.
- **Class II:** Person has little or no limitation in performing day-to-day activities (e.g., dressing, going to the bathroom, showering). However, the person gets tired and winded when climbing a couple flights of stairs or walking uphill.
- **Class III:** Person has marked limitation in performing normal activities. Activities (e.g., dressing, going to the bathroom, showering) leave him tired or out of breath.
- **Class IV:** Person is uncomfortable, tired, and winded even at rest.

How Is Heart Failure Treated?

Managing diet and exercise (see chapter 6) are the key components of heart failure treatment at home. However, there are other important components that all work together to keep the heart functioning as well as possible:

- Medicines such as beta blockers, angiotensin-converting enzyme inhibitors, angiotensin receptor neprilysin inhibitors, and so on (see chapter 7) strengthen the heart muscles and prevent worsening of the heart condition.
- Diuretics or water pills help clear the fluid from the ankles and legs to decrease swelling. Clearing the fluid from the lungs improves breathing.
- Cardiac rehabilitation, a structured exercise program, improves the activity level of heart failure people (reviewed later in this chapter).
- If the person does not improve despite these treatments, a left ventricular assist device and/or heart transplantation (reviewed later in this chapter) may be considered for eligible people.

How Can I Care for the Person with Heart Failure at Home?

Though the diagnosis of heart failure can evoke despondency and resignation, it is important to remember that, with proper care at home and appropriate treatment, the person can have excellent quality of life for a number of years.

The doctor will impress upon the person and caregiver the importance of diet, fluid intake, exercise, blood pressure control, and medicines.

- Dietary choices: Limiting salt intake is a key component of controlling heart failure. Increased salt intake leads to retention of fluid in the body, which leads to swelling of the legs, cough, shortness of breath, and fatigue. Refer to chapter 6 to learn more about monitoring and controlling salt intake.
- Exercise: Daily exercise helps prevent heart conditions. It is equally good for people with heart failure. Routine exercise strengthens the heart and body muscles. It also sends positive signals to the brain. Cardiac rehabilitation is an excellent way to increase the person's confidence in their exercise ability. You should play the role of a cheerleader and encourage the person to exercise routinely. See chapter 6 for details about exercise in heart disease.
- Daily weight: Keeping a log of daily weight helps detect fluid retention before the person has symptoms of heart failure. Early detection and treatment may avoid a worsening condition and hospitalization. See chapter 6 for details about managing weight, especially fluid weight.
- Controlling blood pressure: Blood pressure is the force against which the heart has to pump blood. Normal blood pressure is *around* 120/80 mm, but minor fluctuations are common. However, high blood pressure means the heart has to pump against a greater opposing force. By controlling blood pressure, the workload on the heart is controlled. The person must take all blood pressure medicines and keep a log of daily blood pressure to help ensure that the heart is not subjected to an unnecessary workload. See chapter 6 for details.
- Taking medicines: The doctor and health care team can prescribe the right medicines, but it is all for nothing if the person does not follow the instructions or take the medicines. You need to ensure that the person takes his medicine regularly. Buy a pillbox with a different section for each day of the week, and keep it filled. Use the alarm on the phone as a reminder to take the medicine on time. Keeping a current list of medicines, refilling medicines in time, and working with the health care team to adjust medicines according to the person's condition will help the person avoid hospitalization.

What Is the Outlook for People with Heart Failure?

Longevity and quality of life vary by the person. Those with less severe heart failure, when they are well cared for by caregivers at home, are treated with medicines, and follow guidance from the health care team, can have a long, high-quality life. People with advanced heart failure and many other medical problems and those who do not follow the recommendations of the health care team may have a lower life expectancy.

What Other Steps May Be Taken for People with Heart Failure?

In addition to medicines, people with heart failure may undergo the following procedures:

- Coronary artery bypass surgery: In people with blocked coronary arteries, coronary bypass surgery can improve pumping function of the heart. See details later in this chapter.
- Heart valve repair or replacement: If the heart failure is due to a damaged heart valve, surgery to repair or replace this valve may improve the pumping ability of the heart.
- Implantable cardioverter defibrillator (ICD) implantation: ICDs help prevent death due to fatal arrhythmias common in people with heart failure. In some people, a special type of ICD called a cardiac resynchronization therapy device may be implanted to improve exercise capacity and prevent death from fatal arrhythmias. See details later in this chapter.
- Left ventricular assist device: If medicines and procedures do not alleviate symptoms, this battery-powered mechanical pump can be implanted in *eligible* people to help the weak heart pump adequate blood to the body. See details later in this chapter.
- Heart transplantation: After all other treatment options have been tried, replacing a weak heart with a healthy donor heart may be the only way to increase survival and improve quality of life in *eligible* people. See details later in this chapter.

DISEASES OF THE HEART VALVES

Aortic Stenosis

In this condition, the aortic valve, located between the left ventricle and aorta, narrows and does not open fully (see figure 5.1). As a result, not enough blood flows from the left ventricle into the aorta and the rest of the body. Aortic stenosis is caused by a calcium buildup in the aortic valve due to old age, kidney disease, or radiation to the chest. It is diagnosed using echocardiography (reviewed later in this chapter).

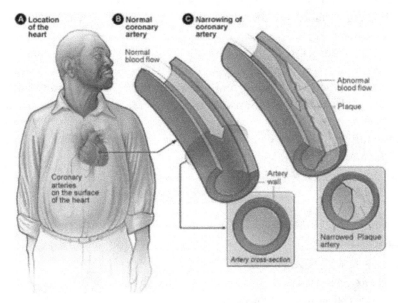

Figure 5.1. In coronary artery disease, the most common heart condition, the coronary arteries that supply blood to the heart muscle are narrowed and blood flow decreases. *National Heart, Lung, and Blood Institute, National Institutes of Health, US Department of Health and Human Services*

In the early stages of the disease, the person may have no symptoms. However, when there is concerning narrowing of the valve, or severe aortic stenosis, the brain receives less blood flow, resulting in dizziness. The heart receives less blood flow, resulting in chest pain, and the body receives less blood flow, resulting in fatigue and shortness of breath. If untreated, the heart muscle weakens, and heart failure ensues. Treatment consists of replacement of the aortic valve, either through open heart surgery or a pinhole surgery through the groin.

Mitral Valve Regurgitation

In this condition, the mitral valve, located between the left atrium and the left ventricle, does not close completely. As a result, blood leaks from the left ventricle back into the left atrium rather than flowing freely into the aorta. Such leakiness, or mitral regurgitation, may be caused by calcium buildup in the mitral valve, a defective mitral valve, enlargement of the left ventricle, infection of the mitral valve, heart attack, or another condition.

Mitral regurgitation is detected using echocardiography (reviewed later in this chapter).

In the early stages of the disease, the person may not have symptoms. However, in severe mitral regurgitation, the body does not receive enough blood from the heart, resulting in shortness of breath, fatigue, and swelling of the ankles and feet. If untreated, the heart muscle weakens, and heart failure ensues. Treatment consists of replacement or repair of the mitral valve through surgery. Alternatively, a pinhole surgery called a mitral valve clip can be performed.

CARDIOMYOPATHY

Cardiomyopathy is any condition that weakens the heart's pumping capacity. Cardiomyopathy may be caused by:

- one or more heart attacks,
- damaged heart valves,
- a virus affecting heart muscles,
- long-term untreated high blood pressure,
- untreated rapid heartbeats for weeks,
- alcohol abuse,
- drug abuse,
- cancer-related medicines weakening the heart muscle,
- other conditions affecting heart muscles (e.g., hypertrophic cardiomyopathy), or
- inflammation of the heart muscle, or myocarditis.

DISEASES AFFECTING THE CORONARY ARTERY

Coronary Artery Disease

This is the most common heart condition, in which the coronary arteries that supply blood to the heart muscle are narrowed due to blockage. These blockages are caused by cholesterol-containing deposits (plaque) and inflammation in the arteries. These plaques build up over years and decades. The arteries gradually narrow, and the flow of oxygen-rich blood to the heart muscle decreases. Such a decrease in blood flow may not have an impact initially, but as the blockages grow blood flow continues to decrease and then the person experiences chest pain (angina) or shortness of breath with exertion (see chapter 2).

With further narrowing, these symptoms appear with minimal exertion and even at rest. People are evaluated with an exercise stress test and cardiac catheterization (reviewed later in this chapter) to look for blockages (narrowing) in the coronary arteries. Depending on the pattern and severity of blockages, medicines, stents, or bypass surgery may be recommended. Medicines such as aspirin, beta blockers, angiotensin-converting enzyme inhibitors, or isosorbide (see chapter 7) may be prescribed. If the person continues to have symptoms despite these medicines, angioplasty or bypass surgery (reviewed later in this chapter) could be the next step.

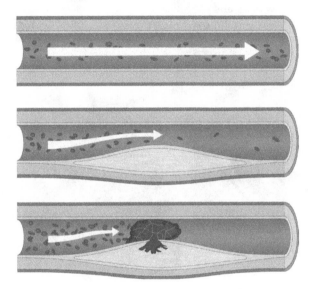

Figure 5.2. If the thin lining covering a cholesterol plaque is damaged, a blood clot forms on top of this minor plaque within hours. The clot completely blocks the coronary artery and cuts off the blood supply, leading to a heart attack. © *DigitalVision Vectors/Getty Images Plus/wetcake*

Heart Attack

As opposed to the gradual narrowing of the coronary arteries mentioned previously, if the thin lining covering a cholesterol plaque is damaged, a rapid reaction takes place. Within hours, a blood clot forms on top of this minor plaque. The clot completely blocks the coronary artery and cuts off the blood supply. This leads to a heart attack, or myocardial infarction. If it is not treated immediately, the heart muscle that depended on that artery for blood supply is damaged permanently. The damaged muscle is replaced by scar tissue and does not pump blood efficiently.

Symptoms of Heart Attack

Heart attack symptoms vary from person to person and can be different in men and women, but most common symptoms are:

- sudden chest pain at rest,
- shortness of breath,
- left arm or jaw pain, and
- nausea and vomiting (in some cases).

Heart Attack

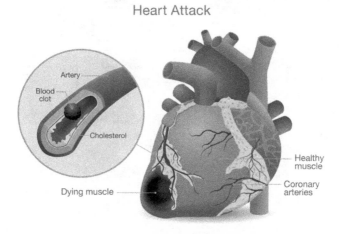

Figure 5.3. Symptoms of a heart attack vary, but the most common are sudden chest pain at rest, shortness of breath, left arm or jaw pain, and nausea and vomiting. © iStock/Getty Images Plus/solar22; © iStock/ Getty Images Plus/ digitalskillet

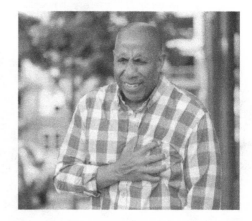

Anyone who has above symptoms must go to the emergency department, where they undergo electrocardiography. If a diagnosis of heart attack is made, emergency angioplasty done in time can restore the blood flow in the coronary artery, thereby salvaging the heart muscle. Additionally, people are treated with aspirin, beta blockers, angiotensin-converting enzyme inhibitors, antiplatelet medicines, or isosorbide (chapter 7).

DISEASES AFFECTING THE ELECTRICAL SYSTEM OF THE HEART

The heart must beat sixty to one hundred times a minute to get enough oxygen-rich blood to the rest of the body. A normal heart produces electrical activity in the sinoatrial node to meet this requirement and start the heartbeat. From here, the electrical activity spreads to the two upper chambers and then to the atrioventricular junction, a bridge between the upper and lower chambers. After a minor delay on this bridge, the electricity spreads to the lower chamber. The spread of the electrical signal then initiates mechanical contraction of the heart chambers. So the upper chambers get the electrical signal and contract first. Moments later, the lower chamber receives the electrical impulses and contracts. The upper and lower chambers contract (beat) one after another in a rhythmic, coordinated manner sixty to one hundred times a minute (hence the corresponding pulse rate of sixty to one hundred a minute). The contraction (squeezing) of the left lower chamber provides oxygen-rich blood throughout the body.

Slow Heartbeat

Under certain circumstances, fewer beats are produced. This happens under one of two conditions:

- The sinoatrial node slows and produces an inadequate number of heartbeats.
- The atrioventricular junction between the upper and lower chambers is damaged, so it cannot send each beat from the upper chamber to the lower chamber.

If the sinoatrial node is damaged, and the heart does not produce enough heartbeats, or the atrioventricular node is damaged and cannot convey electrical activity to the lower chambers, there are insufficient heartbeats and oxygen supply to the body. Such damage can be caused by advanced age, surgery, kidney problems, and, rarely, infections.

Slow Heartbeat Symptoms

- excessive fatigue,
- shortness of breath,
- decreased exercise capacity, and
- daytime sleepiness.

People with slow heartbeats and related symptoms need evaluation of any reversible cause. If none are found or the condition continues despite eliminating the cause, the person will need a pacemaker (reviewed later in this chapter).

Fast Heartbeat

Another type of electrical problem occurs when the heart rate is abnormally high. Such a condition is called tachycardia. Tachycardia can be the result of supraventricular tachycardia (SVT) or atrial fibrillation, which start from the top chambers of the heart (atria), or the result of ventricular tachycardia or ventricular fibrillation (VT/VF), which start from the bottom chambers of the heart (ventricles).

SVT

SVT is an abnormal rhythm from the top chamber of the heart that causes symptoms such as:

- fluttering in the chest,
- palpitations,
- racing heartbeat,
- chest pain,
- shortness of breath,
- lightheadedness or dizziness, or
- near-fainting or fainting.

SVT is caused by an abnormal circuit in the heart. SVT is diagnosed using electrocardiography, a Holter monitor, or an event monitor (reviewed later in this chapter). SVT can be treated with medicines such as beta blockers and calcium channel blockers (see chapter 7). Alternatively, ablation can be performed to cure this condition (reviewed later in this chapter).

Atrial Fibrillation

This condition is a rapid, irregular rhythm from the upper chamber of the heart. Many people have no symptoms. Others feel:

- palpitations or fluttering of the heart,
- rapid heartbeat,
- shortness of breath,
- lightheadedness,
- dizziness, or
- extreme fatigue.

Atrial fibrillation may be caused by:

- advanced age,
- high blood pressure,
- heart valve problems,
- weak heart muscles,
- overactive thyroid,
- lung diseases such as chronic obstructive pulmonary disease or emphysema,
- infection,
- recent surgery, or
- sleep apnea.

People with atrial fibrillation are at high risk for stroke. Blood thinners (e.g., warfarin, Eliquis, Xarelto, Pradaxa) (see chapter 7) are used to decrease this risk. The heart rate in atrial fibrillation is controlled with beta blockers, calcium channel blockers, or, rarely, digoxin. Many people can prevent episodes of atrial fibrillation with medicines such as flecainide, propafenone (Rythmol), sotalol (Betapace, Sorine), amiodarone (Cordarone, Pacerone), or dofetilide (Tikosyn). If medicines cannot control symptoms of atrial fibrillation or the person develops side effects from medicines, ablation may be performed (reviewed later in this chapter).

Abnormal Heart Rhythms from the Ventricles, or VT/VF

This potentially fatal rhythm is caused by heart attacks, weak heart muscles, congestive heart failure, and rare genetic conditions. These rhythms disrupt the normal pumping of the blood and can quickly become life threatening. In these situations, the person may collapse within seconds. Without emergency care, he may die within minutes. Emergency treatment includes cardiopulmonary resuscitation and shocks to the heart from a device called an automated external defibrillator. After resuscitation, the person is stabilized in the hospital and may receive an implantable defibrillator (reviewed later in this chapter).

TESTS

Echocardiogram

An echocardiogram, also called an echo or transthoracic echocardiogram, uses ultrasound to create images of the heart. It is a painless, noninvasive process.

What Does an Echocardiogram Show?

An echocardiogram produces pictures of the heart that show the size of its different chambers, motion of the heart muscles, and overall pumping action. It also shows details of the heart valves.

When Will the Doctor Prescribe an Echocardiogram?

A doctor suggests an echocardiogram when she wants to look at:

- the overall pumping function of the heart,
- the pumping function of different regions of the heart muscle, and
- any leaks or narrowing in the valves of the heart.

Why a Doctor May Recommend an Echocardiogram

- symptoms such as shortness of breath, dizziness, passing out, and swelling of the legs to assess for weakness of the heart;
- a change in symptoms in people with weakness of the heart (cardiomyopathy);
- a new heart murmur;
- a change in symptoms after a murmur is identified;

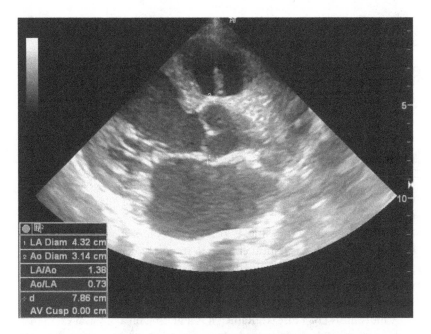

Figure 5.4. Sample echocardiogram. An echocardiogram produces pictures of the heart that show the size of its different chambers, motion of the heart muscles, and overall pumping action. It also shows details of the heart valves. *J Shah, MD*

- a change in a previously identified murmur;
- part of a periodic assessment after a valve leak or narrowing noted on an initial echocardiogram;
- part of periodic assessment after valve replacement (seven years after aortic valve replacement and five years after mitral valve replacement);
- possible infection of the heart valve;
- part of an evaluation of the effects of certain chemotherapy medicines on heart function;
- suspicion of fluid around the heart;
- advanced lung disease, if it may have affected the heart;
- unexplained stroke or mini-stroke;
- a new heart rhythm problem;
- high blood pressure; or
- chest pain that could indicate a heart attack.

The Doctor Said She Wants to Get an Echocardiogram to Assess the Pumping of the Heart. Why?

Shortness of breath, new unexplained fatigue, dizziness, or swelling of the legs could be due to weak pumping of the heart. The doctor may order an echocardiogram to help identify the cause of these symptoms.

The Doctor Said She Heard a Heart Murmur and Wants to Order an Echocardiogram. Why?

A murmur is a sound the doctor heard when listening to the heart with a stethoscope. A murmur indicates that the heart valve may be leaking or narrowing.

The doctor needs to get more information in order to decide if the valve leaking or narrowing is critical enough to merit medicines or surgery or is just something to monitor. The decision depends on the location and severity of the problem. To get this information, the doctor needs to check the valves via an echocardiogram.

A murmur is not a disease. Rather, it is a finding on a physical exam that indicates a possible problem with the heart valves. If the echocardiogram shows no valve problems, there is no reason to worry about the murmur because a murmur by itself does not indicate a heart condition. One does not have to carry the diagnosis of murmur. Think of it as feeling feverish and using a thermometer. If the thermometer does not show increased body temperature, there is no fever.

Are There Any Risks from the Procedure?

An echocardiogram is a noninvasive procedure with low risk.

How Should We Prepare for the Procedure?

Echocardiography is generally performed in a cardiologist's office or a hospital. Because it is noninvasive, no special precautions or preparations are needed. People can usually eat and drink normally and take all their regular medicines as usual before the procedure.

What Happens During the Procedure?

If you have had an ultrasound for a baby or were with a pregnant woman for the ultrasound of her baby, an echocardiogram will remind you of that.

Once signed in, the technician brings the person into the room where the procedure will be performed. The person may be asked to undress from the waist up and wear a gown.

Occasionally, an IV line is started in the forearm. The person is asked to lie on the bed, and the lights are dimmed to allow the technician to see the monitor better during the procedure.

The technician places sticky patches and gel on the chest. Then he uses a wand-like device called a transducer to take ultrasound pictures of the heart. The person may feel extra pressure when the technician tries to get a better look at some parts of the heart. The technician asks the person to lie on the back or left side at different stages of the procedure.

The person may be asked to hold their breath for a moment to allow the technician to get certain pictures of the heart.

During the process, there may be some swooshing sounds from the machine, which is completely normal. Depending on the reason for the echocardiogram, the technician may inject saline into a vein through an IV line. In other cases, he may inject a special ultrasound dye through the IV line to get better images of the heart. All images are recorded for the cardiologist to evaluate and make a diagnosis.

The test takes thirty to sixty minutes. After the test, the technician wipes the gel off the chest and may give the person a paper or cloth towel to further clean up the chest. The person is then asked to change back into regular clothes.

What Happens After the Echocardiogram?

The person can resume normal activities after getting an echocardiogram. Expect a phone call from the doctor about the results of the echocardiogram within a week or so. Sometimes the doctor chooses to discuss the results during the next office visit.

What Will the Results of the Echocardiogram Tell Us?

When the doctor talks about the echocardiogram results, expect to hear about:

- the heart's pumping action;
- any parts of heart muscle that are not moving well;
- any valve leaks;
- any narrowing of valves and whether it is mild, moderate, or severe;

- whether the doctor recommends a follow-up echocardiogram;
- whether the doctor recommends medicine changes based on the results;
- whether the doctor recommends any more procedures (such as cardiac catheterization);
- whether the doctor recommends surgery; and
- whether the echocardiogram ruled out any conditions and whether there is a need for another test for diagnosis of the symptoms.

What Questions Should I Ask the Doctor When an Echocardiogram Is Ordered?

It is important to understand why the doctor ordered the echocardiogram and how the results will affect what is done next. If the person had an echocardiogram recently, it may be worth asking how much new information the next echocardiogram will add.

What Will the Echocardiogram Results Show?

The echocardiogram results give information about:

- Thickness of heart muscle: People with high blood pressure have thickened heart muscle. Some rare genetic conditions may also cause thickening.
- Size of the heart: An enlarged heart can be seen on an echocardiogram.
- Pumping function: The heart pumping function is given as a number called ejection fraction. A normal heart has an ejection fraction of 55 percent to 70 percent. A heart that pumps less than 55 percent is abnormal.
- Wall motion abnormality: Echocardiograms can show if certain parts of the heart muscle do not move as briskly as other parts, indicating a wall motion abnormality. If the person has had a heart attack, it may show up as abnormal wall motion in the affected area. Another major cause is a narrowing of the artery supplying that wall (part) of the heart muscle. In this case, the doctor may prescribe cardiac catheterization to check the arteries.
- Valve function: An echocardiogram is the final word on the health of the heart valves. Valves can be either leaky or narrowed. The severity of valve leaks and valve narrowing is graded as mild, moderate, or severe. Mild and moderate leaking or narrowed valves do not need to be replaced; instead, the doctor may give medicines and monitor the valve over time. However, severe leaks or narrowing may require repair or replacement. In this case, the person may need to see a surgeon.

- Holes in the heart: Very infrequently an echocardiogram detects holes in the heart that need to be fixed.
- Fluid or blood clots: Sometimes fluid builds up around the heart and shows up on the echocardiogram. Rarely, clots and tumors are found. Clots in the heart can move to the brain and cause a stroke, so they need to be addressed.

Holter and Event Monitors

What Are Holter and Event Monitors?

Holter and event monitors are portable, battery-operated devices that record electrocardiography (EKG) continuously. The person is connected to the monitor for one or more days to record the EKG while he performs his daily activities. It is a noninvasive test performed when the person has fleeting fluttering of the heart, skipped beats, lightheadedness, or occasional episodes of passing out, and the doctor suspects that brief abnormal heart rhythms are the cause. Wearing a monitor 24/7 for days or weeks records these abnormal rhythms and helps the doctor diagnose the problem.

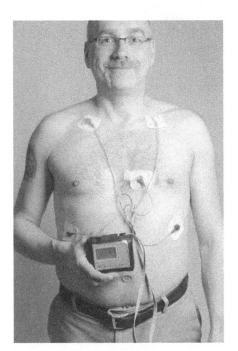

Figure 5.5. Holter and event monitors are portable, battery-operated devices that record electrocardiography continuously. © E+/Getty Images Plus/marcduf

What Is the Device Like?

The Holter monitor has three parts: (1) three to five soft, sticky, silver-dollar-sized patches, or electrodes, attached to different spots on the chest; (2) wires connected to each electrode; and (3) a pager-sized gadget connected to the wires. This gadget can be clipped to the waistband or worn around the neck.

The event monitor also has three parts: (1) three electrodes; (2) wires connected to each electrode; and (3) a smartphone-sized gadget connected to the wires. Although many event monitors look similar to Holter monitors, more devices are coming to the market with different designs.

Event monitors have a button that the person presses to indicate symptoms. The device stores the EKG at that time and helps the doctor connect the symptoms to the heart rhythm and diagnose the problem. It is critical that the person presses the button so as to make recording of the EKG at the time of the symptoms.

These devices can be worn under clothing so that the person can wear it in public without attracting attention.

Why Did the Doctor Order This Test?

Holter monitors continuously record the heart rhythm for twenty-four to forty-eight hours. The doctor orders this for people who experience these symptoms daily:

- fluttering of the heart, or palpitations;
- skipped beats;
- excessive fatigue;
- lightheadedness or dizziness; or
- passing out, or syncope.

It may also be ordered if the doctor suspects:

- a low heart rate,
- a temporary drop in heartbeats,
- extra beats, or
- rapid heartbeats.

If the person has fleeting symptoms once or twice a week, the doctor may suspect a transient abnormal heart rhythm and order an event monitor. When the person presses the button to indicate symptoms, the device stores the EKG at that time. The doctor then connects the symptoms with the heart rhythm problem recorded on the EKG and diagnoses the person's condition.

These devices are also programmed to automatically store any abnormal rhythms. So, even if the person is unaware, the device detects, records, and stores the abnormal rhythm. Some devices can transmit the abnormal EKG right away to the device company. If the recording is deemed critical, company staff call the person and send the abnormal EKG tracing immediately to the doctor.

What Questions Should I Ask the Doctor If She Prescribes a Monitor?

- What symptoms will the monitor address?
- How long is the monitoring period?
- What will the test tell us about the person's heart?
- Will the results lead to other tests? New medicines? Procedures?
- If the symptoms are not too frequent or bothersome, does the person still need this test?
- What if the symptoms do not occur while the person wears the monitor?

What Does the Monitor Show?

Holter monitors make continuous EKG recordings for twenty-four or forty-eight hours. Every heartbeat is recorded to inform the doctor about:

- minimum heart rate;
- maximum heart rate;
- any extra beats (i.e., premature atrial contractions or premature ventricular contractions) and, if so, the number over twenty-four or forty-eight hours;
- any abnormal rapid heartbeats (i.e., tachycardias such as supraventricular tachycardia or atrial fibrillation); and
- any abnormal slow heartbeats (i.e., bradycardia or missed heartbeats).

As the name indicates, event monitors monitor events. If the person has palpitations or a racing heart, he can press the button to record and store the EKG during the event. The event monitor also automatically records abnormal heartbeats even when the person is not aware of them.

Do These Monitors Pose Any Risks?

These monitoring devices cause no pain. A few people have allergic reaction to the electrodes. Otherwise, it is a noninvasive test with few negative effects.

These monitors are not water resistant and should not get wet. The person cannot shower or swim while wearing one. Some monitors can be removed and reattached after taking a shower. The technician who initially connects the device can give guidance on showering during monitoring.

Most people have no trouble sleeping with the monitor connected to them. The person and you should ensure that the wires do not accidentally disconnect at night.

How Should the Person Prepare?

The person is given an appointment to get the monitor connected. No specific preparation is needed. There is no need to withhold medicine or fast beforehand.

What Happens During Monitoring?

During the appointment, a trained technician brings the person to a room to connect the monitor. The person removes his clothes from the waist up and any jewelry that may interfere with attaching the electrodes. Because body hair can interfere with proper attachment of the electrodes, the technician may shave some hair before connecting the electrodes, wires, and monitor.

The technician explains how to take care of the device. The technician may clip the device to your waist belt. If the location of the device is not comfortable, ask for alternative places to carry the device. Ask if the batteries need to be changed and, if so, what kind of batteries should be used and how to change them.

The technician gives a symptom "diary" or paper to write down symptoms such as palpitations, skipped beats, and dizziness during monitoring. The person should record these symptoms and the activity, food intake, exercise, or stress level at the time. This step is critical. The doctor uses the diary to correlate the symptoms to the EKG and diagnose the person's condition. If the person does not provide an accurate record, the test will not help the doctor diagnose the condition.

The person should avoid activities that could get the electrodes or device wet. The person can perform all other activities. The person and you should learn how to reattach the wires and electrodes if they fall off. Avoid metal detectors, magnets, electric blankets, and electric razors and toothbrushes to prevent device interference. Cell phones should be kept at least six inches from the monitor. Ask about any other electrical gadgets to avoid during monitoring.

An event monitor is connected to the person in the same manner. However, the recording of the symptoms is extremely critical. Event monitors have a button that the person or caregiver presses during palpitations, skipped beats, dizziness, or fluttering to record and store the EKG.

The doctor connects the symptoms and the EKG based on this recording. Successful monitoring depends on the person making appropriate recordings, so it is important to understand how to indicate symptoms. If you are unclear about this, ask the technician to explain again. It may be worth practicing before leaving the office. The technician tells you how to return the device at the end of monitoring.

What Happens After Monitoring?

For Holter monitors, after the monitoring period, return the device as instructed and submit the symptom diary. Holter monitors are generally returned to the doctor's clinic or the office where they were connected. The technician cannot give the results immediately. She downloads the information from the monitor and compiles a report for the doctor. The doctor then assesses and correlates the symptoms with the EKG to diagnose the person's condition. She prepares a final report based on these findings.

For event monitors, return the event monitor to the doctor's office or mail it to the monitoring company as directed. The device company and/or the doctor's office monitors the EKG recording. If the findings are concerning, the device may transmit it immediately to the monitoring company. The person receives a phone call in such a situation. If no critical findings appear during monitoring, the doctor gets a complete report of the symptoms and the EKG after monitoring is complete. She assesses the report, correlates the person's symptoms with the EKG during symptoms, and diagnoses the person's condition. She discusses it with the person at the next visit.

What Can We Expect to Learn from the Results?

The monitor can detect if a heart rhythm problem is responsible for any of these symptoms:

- palpitations,
- racing of the heart,

- dizziness,
- episodes of passing out (syncope),
- fluttering of the heart, or
- excessive, unexpected fatigue.

If so, treatment of these abnormal rhythms, or arrhythmias, with medicine will help resolve the symptoms. Sometimes, procedures like ablation
(reviewed later in this chapter) or cardioversion may be performed to treat
these arrhythmias.

The device may also detect silent arrhythmias. Depending on the type
of arrhythmia, the doctor may treat it or leave it alone. In rare instances
in which the silent episodes herald an ominous outcome, the doctor may
choose to treat preemptively despite a lack of symptoms.

If the person does not have abnormal heart rhythms or symptoms during
monitoring, the doctor cannot make the diagnosis. She may then recommend a one-month event monitor.

What Questions Should I Ask the Doctor About the Results?

That depends on the purpose of the monitor. If the monitor was prescribed
for specific symptoms, the key questions are:

- Did we capture the EKG at the time of the symptoms?
- If so, are the symptoms related to an abnormal heart rhythm?
- If so, how do we treat it?
- If the symptoms are unrelated to heart rhythm problems, how do we
  identify their cause?

Sometimes, fleeting symptoms may not occur during monitoring. In that
case, it is important to discuss if longer-term monitoring could identify the
cause of the symptoms.

If the monitor was done to check for a silent rhythm problem, ask if arrhythmias were noted on the monitor. If so, ask what changes are recommended as a result.

Exercise Stress Test
What Is a Stress Test?

A cardiac stress test, also called an exercise stress test or treadmill test, deter-
mines if there is sufficient blood flow to the heart muscles. The heart works

harder during exercise. In order to work harder, the heart needs increased blood flow. If the arteries supplying blood to the heart (coronary arteries) are narrowed, the heart muscle cannot get enough blood. This causes chest pain, electrocardiogram (EKG) changes, or changes in blood pressure. If these changes occur during an exercise stress test, they suggest narrowing (blockages) in the coronary arteries.

Why Did the Doctor Suggest a Stress Test?

Stress tests look for narrowing (blockages) in the coronary arteries. If symptoms such as chest pain, shortness of breath, and excessive fatigue suggest such narrowing, the doctor recommends a stress test.

Occasionally, it is recommended prior to a high-risk surgery to ensure safety of the surgery.

How Should the Person Prepare for a Stress Test?

The doctor's office provides instructions before the test. It is a good idea to write them down. The person may be asked to:

- not eat or drink after midnight the day of the test;
- avoid caffeine for thirty-six hours before certain types of stress tests;
- wear or bring comfortable clothes and walking shoes;
- stop using beta blockers (e.g., metoprolol, carvedilol, atenolol) before the procedure;
- bring any inhalers used for breathing problems to the test;
- inform the team about all medicines used, especially inhalers and beta blockers; and
- avoid using any oil, lotion, or cream on the skin the day of a nuclear stress test.

What Happens During a Stress Test?

The technician places soft, sticky patches called electrodes on the person's chest. The technician may shave the chest hair so that the electrodes stick better. The electrodes are then connected to wires, which in turn are connected to an EKG machine. The technician places a blood pressure cuff on the arm.

The doctor or an assistant asks questions about the person's medical history and performs a quick physical exam. Then the person gets on the treadmill or exercise bike to start the test.

The work that the person has to perform is increased gradually. During this process, the EKG, blood pressure, and heart rate are checked. The exercise continues until the person reaches a certain heart rate. If she has symptoms of severe chest pain, shortness of breath, dizziness, or fatigue, inform the technician. If the technician notices changes in heart rhythm or blood pressure, she may stop the test.

Once the test is complete, the treadmill is stopped, and the person is asked to stand still for a few seconds and then lie on a bed. The team continues to monitor for abnormalities on the EKG and blood pressure. After a few minutes, when the person's heart rate has slowed, the electrode patches are removed, and the person can go home and resume normal activities.

Nuclear Stress Test

Doctors often recommend a stress test with radioactive dye. In this case, a technician injects radioactive dye before the exercise and places the person in a nuclear camera to get images of the heart.

The person exercises on a treadmill or bike. The technician injects dye once again at the peak of exercise. After exercise, she takes another set of heart images under the nuclear camera. The before-and-after pictures of the heart help the doctor detect any narrowing (blockages) in the coronary arteries.

Stress Echocardiogram

Occasionally, instead of radioactive dye, the doctor may do an echocardiogram before and after the exercise. This test further helps to detect blockages in the coronary arteries.

Chemical Stress Test or Pharmacologic Stress Test

If the person cannot exercise, the doctor may order a chemical stress test. In this case, the technician injects radioactive dye when the person is at rest and gets pictures of the heart. Then he gives the person medicine to increase the blood flow to the heart. The technician then injects the radioactive dye and takes pictures again. As before, the doctor reviews the before-and-after pictures to identify any narrowing (blockages) in the heart arteries.

The medicine used during the test may briefly make the person feel flushed or short of breath. However, this sensation fades quickly.

Why Is an Echocardiogram or Radioactive Dye Needed Along with the Exercise Stress Test?

The EKG part of the stress test is helpful, but it may miss coronary artery narrowing (blockages) in some people. A radioactive dye or echocardiogram-based stress test decreases the chance of missing these blockages.

The Person Was Able to Walk on the Treadmill for More Than Ten Minutes. Is That a Good Sign?

This is an excellent sign. Exercise duration is one of the strongest predictors of future health outcomes. The longer the person can keep going on the treadmill, the less likely he is to have a heart attack in the near future.

What Should I Watch for After a Stress Test?

Aftercare for an exercise stress test is similar to aftercare for exercise. So, if the person is tired after the stress test, he should rest and stay hydrated. If the person feels lightheaded immediately after, inform the technician. Once a person leaves the hospital or clinic, he is unlikely to have further problems.

If a chemical rather than an exercise stress test is performed, nothing further should occur because the medicine washes out of the system within seconds to minutes.

How Will the Doctor Report the Stress Test Results?

A stress test result reports how long the person exercised and the effect of exercise on heart rate, blood pressure, and the EKG.

A nuclear stress test and stress echocardiogram also report on the pumping function of the heart. The doctor typically informs the person whether the stress test was normal or abnormal.

What Will We Find Out When the Doctor Discusses the Stress Test Results?

When the doctor discusses stress test results, expect to hear about:

- exercise time;
- concerns about heart rate, blood pressure, or EKG during exercise;
- any concerns about blockages in the coronary arteries; and
- in case of a nuclear stress test or stress echocardiogram, the pumping function of the heart (ejection fraction).

What Are the Next Steps After the Stress Test?

If the stress test was performed for clearance for surgery, a normal stress test is a go-ahead for surgery.

If the test was performed to assess symptoms such as chest pain and shortness of breath and it was normal, the symptoms are not related to narrowing (blockages) in the coronary arteries. The doctor will recommend other tests to assess the symptoms.

If the test was abnormal, it suggests blockages in the coronary arteries. In this case, the doctor may recommend a coronary angiogram, also known as cardiac catheterization. This is the best way to identify any blockages in the heart arteries. On occasion, the doctor may alternatively choose a special computed tomographic (CT) scan to detect any blockages.

If the Stress Test Is Normal, Does It Mean That the Person Will Not Have a Heart Attack?

A normal stress test tells the doctor that the chances of a heart attack are low but not zero. Sometimes people die of a heart attack after having a normal stress test. However, this does not mean that stress tests are unreliable. It only means that these rare cases still occur. A normal stress test is usually a fairly reliable test but is not a guarantee against heart attacks in the future.

The Person Has Had Heart Disease and Bypass Surgery. Should a Stress Test Be Performed Every Year?

No. Unless new symptoms appear, the person does not need a routine annual stress test.

Cardiac Catheterization

What Is Cardiac Catheterization?

Cardiac catheterization, also known as a cath or coronary angiogram, is the gold standard test to look for narrowing (blockages) in the coronary arteries. In this procedure, the doctor accesses an artery in an arm or leg. From there, she threads a small, thin, flexible tube called a catheter into the coronary arteries. She then injects dye into the coronary arteries while taking X-ray pictures. The dye flows through the arteries, making them easy to see on X-ray. A blockage in the artery, or stenosis, is visible as a narrowing on the X-ray.

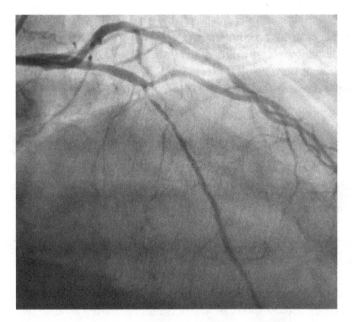

Figure 5.6. Cardiac catheterization showing blockage in coronary artery. Cardiac catheterization, also known as a cath or coronary angiogram, is the gold standard test to look for blockages in the coronary arteries. *J Shah, MD*

When Is Cardiac Catheterization Recommended?

A doctor recommends cardiac catheterization when she suspects complete blockage in the coronary arteries, such as during a heart attack. However, the procedure is most often done when the doctor suspects narrowing of the coronary artery due to the person's symptoms and risk factors. A cardiac catheterization is a standard follow-up test to an abnormal stress test.

How Should the Person Prepare for the Procedure?

The doctor's office gives written instructions about the procedure and calls to provide further instructions. It is a good idea to write down these instructions. The general guidelines in preparation for a cardiac catheterization procedure are:

- Do not eat or drink anything after midnight before the procedure.
- Bring medicine bottles along to the procedure.

- People with diabetes need to understand the doctor's advice about taking any diabetes pills or insulin injections.
- People taking blood thinners (warfarin, Coumadin, Jantoven, Eliquis, Pradaxa, or Xarelto) need to understand the doctor's directions for stopping these medicines.

What Happens at the Hospital Before the Procedure?

You or the person complete paperwork and check in for the cardiac catheterization. Then you and the person are taken to a room in the catheterization lab area, where these steps are taken to prepare for the procedure:

- changing into a patient gown and removing any dentures or jewelry;
- checking the person's blood pressure, pulse, and temperature;
- inserting an intravenous (IV) line into the person's arm and drawing blood for testing;
- shaving the person's groin or arm;
- signing the consent form to give the doctor permission to perform the procedure and use blood products, if needed, during an emergency (the doctor may review the risks and benefits of the procedure and answer any questions);
- verifying information about the person's general health;
- verifying any previous problems the person has had with medicines (if the person has had trouble with anesthesia in the past, advise the staff); and
- using the restroom to empty the bladder or bowel before the procedure.

The person is then taken to the procedure room.

What Happens During the Procedure?

The person is transferred to the catheterization lab for the procedure. He lies down on a special table and is given IV medicine to keep him relaxed and pain-free. He will likely be semi-awake for the procedure.

Staff place soft, sticky patches called electrodes on the person's chest, arms, and legs to monitor the electrocardiogram; prepare the catheterization site; and cover the person in a sterile drape.

The doctor injects local anesthesia near the arm or groin artery to keep the person pain-free.

Once the area is numb, she inserts a needle into the artery and places a plastic tube called a sheath. She passes the catheter through the sheath to the coronary arteries. Once the catheter is well positioned, she injects dye and takes X-ray pictures of the coronary arteries. She takes multiple pictures by positioning the X-ray machine at different locations around the person's body to view the arteries from many angles. On occasion, she may ask the person to take a deep breath or hold his breath.

The doctor may also inject dye into the heart itself and check its pumping. This may cause a flushed, warm sensation throughout the person's body.

The doctor then removes the catheter and may tell the person the results of the procedure. If the person is too sleepy, the doctor may wait to talk about the results. In the meantime, she may discuss the results with you.

If the person needs an angioplasty or stent (reviewed later in this chapter), the doctor may proceed immediately.

What Happens After the Procedure?

The sterile drape is removed, and the person is taken to the recovery room, which may be the same room where he was prepared for the procedure. The plastic sheath that was inserted into the groin or arm is removed.

A staff member applies pressure to the insertion sites. If the groin was used, the person must lie flat for several hours. He can eat and drink at this point.

The time of hospital release depends on the treatment plan, which is based on the results of the procedure.

How Are the Results Reported?

The results of cardiac catheterization are reported as a percentage of stenosis in different coronary arteries (e.g., 40 percent stenosis [narrowing] in the right coronary artery and 30 percent blockage in the left main artery). The pumping function of the heart is reported as an ejection fraction.

Based on the number of narrowed arteries and the degree of narrowing (stenosis), the doctor recommends medicine, angioplasty (with stent), bypass surgery, or a combination of these.

How Are the Results Interpreted?

Stenosis of less than 50 percent in the left main artery and less than 70 percent in other arteries requires treatment with medicine, exercise, and diet. This degree of narrowing is not critical and does not require surgery or stents.

What Questions Should I Ask if the Person Is Recommended for Cardiac Catheterization?

- Which symptoms are we trying to address with cardiac catheterization?
- Could there be other causes of these symptoms?
- Does the person have many risk factors that make blockages likely?
- Can any noninvasive tests be performed before cardiac catheterization?
- If a stress test has been performed, how much of the person's heart is affected by low blood flow?
- If a stress test suggests blockages, can the person try medicine first?
- If you find narrowing (blockages) in the coronary arteries, is the person a candidate for surgery?
- Instead of surgery, can the person start with medical treatment and life-style changes first?
- What are the specific risks from the procedure?

What Are the Risks of the Procedure?

There are many ways to identify blockages in the coronary arteries. Like all invasive procedures, cardiac catheterization has risks. For every one hundred people undergoing this procedure, two have major complications related to it such as:

- heart attack related to the test,
- stroke,
- damage to the heart artery,
- puncture of a wall of the heart and blood seeping outside the heart (tamponade),
- kidney damage,
- infection,
- blood clots, or
- death.

Besides these major complications, minor complications such as these can occur:

- bruising or blood accumulation in the arm or groin,
- damage to the artery of the arm or groin (pseudoaneurysm),
- irregular heart rhythms (arrhythmias), or
- allergic reaction to the IV dye.

How Do I Take Care of the Person After the Procedure?

Before leaving the hospital, get an updated list of medicines to be used. Make sure you understand any new medicine to start and any previous medicines to stop. Make a follow-up appointment.

The person should drink eight to ten glasses of water during the twenty-four hours after the procedure.

The person will have a small bandage on his groin or arm. The next morning, wet the bandage and remove it. Wash this site gently with soap and water once a day for the next five days. Keep it dry the rest of the time.

Do not use creams or lotions on the site. The person should avoid wearing tight clothes for the first week and getting into a hot tub, pool, or lake for seven days.

Watch for bruising around the site, which is normal. It is not unusual to have a quarter-sized lump. However, if the lump increases or is painful, contact the doctor.

The person may feel tired the day after the procedure and should rest and walk around the house for the first two days. He should avoid strenuous activities such as running and golfing for a week and should climb stairs slowly. After the first week, he can gradually be more active.

Do not put pressure on the groin or arm where the procedure was done. If the groin was used, the person should not strain during bowel movements for the first week. He should avoid lifting more than ten pounds or pushing or pulling anything heavy for a week.

Most people can resume driving in one or two days, a desk job in two or three days, and sex in a week.

Calcium Score

A calcium score, also called a heart scan, is a computed tomographic (CT) test to detect blockages (narrowing) in the coronary arteries in people with risk factors for coronary artery disease (CAD) but no symptoms.

Plaques made of calcium, fat, cholesterol, and other materials can clog the coronary arteries. Measurement of the amount of calcium in the coronary artery tells the doctor about blockage.

These blockages appear long before people feel symptoms. Doctors use the calcium score to understand the nature of the blockage and get an early start on treatment.

When Do Doctors Recommend a Calcium Score?

Doctors recommend this test for people with risk factors for CAD such as smoking, diabetes, abnormal cholesterol levels, age older than fifty-five, male sex, and a family history of premature CAD.

A calcium score is also appropriate for people with no symptoms but a 10 percent to 20 percent risk for CAD in the next ten years.

How Can I Find Out the Person's Risk of CAD in the Next Ten Years?

Here is a calculator to help you to assess the risk: cvriskcalculator.com/. If you are in doubt or worried, call your doctor.

When Should a Calcium Score Not Be Performed?

The following people are likely to be harmed more than helped by a calcium score test:

- men younger than forty years and women younger than fifty,
- people with a very low risk of CAD,
- people with a very high risk of CAD,
- people who already know they have CAD,
- people whose doctor has ordered a calcium score as part of preoperative screening,
- people with symptoms that are likely caused by narrowing (blockages) in the heart arteries, and
- people with a previously abnormal heart scan.

What Are the Risks of a Calcium Score?

A heart scan uses X-rays, so the small risk of developing cancer due to X-rays also applies to the calcium score test. The risk of cancer, though very small, increases with each X-ray and scan.

How Should the Person Prepare for the Heart Scan?

Below are some tips to help people prepare for the procedure:

- Avoid caffeine and tobacco in all forms for four hours before the test.
- Avoid wearing jewelry to the test.

- Anticipate changing into a patient gown, and dress accordingly.
- Do not apply powder or lotion to the chest before the test.

What Happens During the Test?

The person is asked to remove any jewelry and change into a gown. She may be given medicine to slow the heart rate and allow the technician to capture better images. Medicine may also be given for anxiety.

Staff place soft, sticky patches called electrodes on the person's chest, and the person is asked to lie on a movable table.

The technician sits in the next room and operates the scanner. During the procedure, he slides the patient table in and out of a tube as needed. Occasionally, the person is asked to hold her breath. The person may hear clicking sounds during the procedure.

After about fifteen minutes, the technician says that the scan is complete and removes the electrodes. The person changes back into her clothes and can resume normal daily activities.

How Does the Doctor Report the Results of the Scan, and What Do They Mean?

A heart scan is reported as a number called the Agatston score. A score of zero to 100 indicates a very low chance of CAD and future risk of a heart attack. A score of more than 400 indicates the presence of CAD and a high future risk of a heart attack.

Alternatively, a score is given as a percentile that indicates a person's calcium score relative to others of the same age and sex. The lower the percentile, the lower the risk of CAD or a heart attack.

What Should We Expect When Discussing the Results with the Doctor?

A doctor will discuss the results of the heart scan with you and the person. Depending on the outcome, he may recommend:

- exercising,
- quitting smoking,
- improving the diet,
- setting weight-loss goals,
- starting statin medicines, or
- further testing of the heart.

The table below may also guide a person in making beneficial lifestyle changes, depending on the Agatston score:

Score	Possible actions
1–100	Quit smoking, eat better, and exercise more.
101–400	Quit smoking, eat better, and exercise more. Further testing may be required.
More than 400	Quit smoking, eat better, and exercise more. Further testing may be required.

Are There Alternatives to a Calcium Score?

Yes. Many other tests can assess the risk of heart disease and heart attacks, including:

- cholesterol test,
- stress test, and
- risk factor assessment.

TREATMENTS

Cardiac Rehabilitation

Cardiac rehabilitation, or cardiac rehab, is an exercise program performed under expert supervision. The program is individualized to the person's medical status and physical fitness. In addition to exercise training, the person receives emotional support and lifestyle education to recover from their heart condition or surgery and increase their activity level. Cardiac rehab also helps people quit smoking, adopt a heart-healthy diet, and adhere to regular medicine use.

What Are the Benefits of Cardiac Rehab?

People who undergo cardiac rehab tend to:

- live longer,
- have a lower chance of cardiac events such as heart attacks and heart surgery,
- have a better quality of life,
- have better physical health,
- have a healthy lifestyle,
- eat a healthy diet,
- have increased energy,

- maintain physical strength and fitness,
- maintain a healthy weight,
- have better blood pressure control,
- have better cholesterol levels,
- use fewer medicines,
- have less stress and depression, and
- be emotionally stable.

Who Decides if the Person Needs Cardiac Rehab?

Cardiac rehab is recommended by the doctor if the person has had:

- heart procedures and surgeries,
- heart attack,
- heart transplant, or
- heart failure.

Unfortunately, a busy doctor may fail to refer the person for this high-impact therapy. As part of the health care team, you should ask the cardiologist or primary care physician if the person would benefit from cardiac rehab. The doctor can make a referral and enroll the person in the program. Depending on the person's heart condition, cardiac rehab may be started a week after release from the hospital. In some cases, the doctor may delay it for a few weeks.

You should go with the person for the initial few sessions and then as many sessions as possible. Together with the rehab team, you will set achievable goals and map the path to achieving them. If there are any obstacles to successful participation in the program, you and the person should mention it. The health care team may be able to help you troubleshoot the problem.

Remember that, although the doctor decides if the person needs cardiac rehab, your and the person's motivation, dedication, and efforts determine if it will succeed. All major insurance plans, as well as Medicare, cover the cost of cardiac rehab, although a copay may be required.

Does Cardiac Rehab Pose Any Risks?

The doctor will recommend cardiac rehab when the person is ready for it. Muscular injuries may occur from physical activity during cardiac rehab. However, performing these activities under supervision is the best way to avoid them.

Occasionally, high blood pressure, a high heart rate, or an abnormal heart rhythm is noted during cardiac rehab. The therapists will address these issues in collaboration with the person's doctors.

What Activities Does the Person Do in Cardiac Rehab?

Cardiac rehab may start in the hospital immediately after a cardiac event or surgery. Most cardiac rehab is carried out in an outpatient clinic three times a week for twelve weeks. In rare cases, it is done at home with a visiting therapist.

The team is made up of experts such as physical therapists, occupational therapists, nurses, nurse educators, dietitians, exercise physiologists, social workers, and counselors. The person will undergo an initial evaluation to determine the goals of cardiac rehab and how to achieve them. The team will determine the risks with exercise based on the person's medical condition, fitness, and individual needs. Although each person's cardiac rehab program is individualized, these are the basic components:

- **Exercise training:** Even if the person has never exercised before, the professionals will teach him proper warm-up and cooldown techniques. They will also teach proper methods of performing low-impact exercises such as walking, jogging, cycling, swimming, or climbing stairs. Muscle-strengthening exercise such as lifting weights or using elastic bands or wall pulleys may be a part of the routine. The physical therapist and exercise physiologist will gradually increase the exercise to improve the person's cardiovascular strength. This will enhance the person's confidence in his ability to perform similar exercises at home. You should observe and plan to help the person replicate these exercises at home.

- **Healthy lifestyle training:** The dietitians, social workers, and counselors will assess the person's risk factors for heart disease and future heart attacks. The person will be guided to eliminate tobacco and alcohol use and maintain a heart-healthy diet and healthy weight. With ample one-on-one time with the professionals, lots of questions about day-to-day activities will be answered during the rehab program. By participating in these activities, you can help reinforce these instructions at home to transition the person to a healthier lifestyle.

- **Coping with stress:** It is not unusual for a person to feel anxious, depressed, and stressed after a cardiac event. Stress has a negative physical and emotional impact. The counselors, as a part of the cardiac rehab team, will help identify ways in which stress can be handled in an effective and healthy manner. They will help the person work through this difficult phase and return to an active life. You can recognize the potential stresses and work with the counselors to make plans to reduce the impact of stress on the person. You can further help the person implement the counselors' and social workers' recommendations.

What Happens When the Cardiac Rehab Program Ends?

The cardiac rehab program will help the person transition to a healthy life-style. The person should continue the exercise routine and heart-healthy diet and remain tobacco-free after the formal cardiac rehab program ends. At the end of the program, you and the person will feel comfortable and confident continuing the exercise program at home or at a local gym.

You take over the role of the counselor as well as physical therapist in mo-tivating the person to carry on healthy habits and manage emotions down the road.

Coronary Artery Bypass Grafting (CABG)

CABG is a surgery in which a healthy artery in the chest or vein from the legs is connected, or grafted, to a blocked coronary artery. The grafted artery or vein goes around, or bypasses, the blocked part of the coronary artery, allowing blood to flow freely to the heart again. Multiple grafts can be done in a single surgery. For example, when grafts are done on all three arteries, it is known as a triple heart bypass.

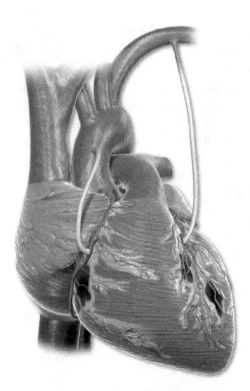

Figure 5.7. Bypassing blocked coronary arteries with coronary artery bypass grafting, a surgery in which a healthy artery in the chest or vein from the legs is connected, or grafted, to a blocked coronary artery. The grafted artery or vein goes around, or bypasses, the blocked part of the coronary artery, allowing blood to flow freely to the heart again. Blausen.com staff (29 August 2014), "Medical gallery of Blausen Medical 2014," *WikiJournal of Medicine* 1 (2), doi:10.15347/WJM/2014.010, ISSN 2002-4436, Wikidata Q44276831

When Does a Person Need CABG?

The decision whether to use medicines vs. medicines and stent vs. medicines and CABG depends on the severity of the narrowing and whether the person has symptoms (e.g., shortness of breath, pain) due to these blockages.

The American College of Cardiology and the American Heart Association recommend CABG to lengthen the person's life, even if there are no symptoms, if there is:

- more than 50 percent narrowing in the left main artery;
- more than 70 percent narrowing in all three coronary arteries;
- more than 70 percent narrowing in the early part of the left anterior descending artery and one more artery especially in people with diabetes;
- more than 70 percent narrowing in two coronary arteries and a very abnormal stress test (a test that monitors heart function during exercise); or
- more than 70 percent narrowing in two coronary arteries and heart pumping function of 35 percent to 50 percent (normal range, 55 percent or higher).

If the doctor believes that the symptoms of chest pain, shortness of breath, or jaw pain are related to narrowing of the coronary artery, he will recommend surgery to relieve symptoms if there is:

- more than 70 percent narrowing in one, two, or three arteries (or 50 percent narrowing in the left main artery combined with more than 70 percent in any of the others) and lifestyle modification and all available medicine-based treatments have not helped relieve symptoms, or
- more than 70 percent narrowing in one, two, or three arteries (or 50 percent blockage in the left main artery), and medicines are not suitable, or the person does not want to take medicine.

What Are the Risks of CABG?

In the United States, the risk of death after bypass surgery ranges from one in one hundred to one in twenty depending on the person's condition and details of the surgery. Other complications include:

- internal bleeding and the need for reoperation (one in twenty-eight surgeries);
- stroke (one in one hundred surgeries);
- infection of the incision site;

- infection in the bloodstream;
- heart attack;
- pneumonia;
- kidney problems (one in forty-three surgeries);
- the need for extended life support or ventilation (one in fourteen surgeries);
- occasional heart rhythm problem called atrial fibrillation;
- cognitive, or mental, decline (one in four surgeries);
- need for a permanent pacemaker; or
- pericardial effusion (fluid around the heart) or pleural effusion (fluid around the lungs) that may make breathing difficult.

People at high risk for these complications are those with:

- age older than eighty years;
- previous cardiac surgery;
- poor heart function; or
- lung problems, diabetes, or kidney problems.

Complication rates vary by hospital, with those performing more than 450 CABGs per year having lower complication rates than those performing fewer than 150 per year.

What Should We Ask the Cardiologist or Cardiac Surgeon Before We Consent to CABG?

- How much of each artery is narrowed (blocked)?
- Do you think the symptoms are related to coronary artery disease?
- If the person has no symptoms, do you recommend the surgery because you believe it will prolong her life?
- Can we try medicine before surgery?
- How many bypass surgeries do you and the hospital perform each year? The more surgeries the surgeon and his team do, the lower the chances of complications. It is important to remember that the rate of death as a result of CABG is much higher in hospitals performing fewer than 150 CABGs per year than in those performing 450 or more CABGs per year. The same is true for the average length of hospital stay and the frequency of further surgery, infection, need for blood transfusion, and other complications.
- Can we wait to decide whether the person wants surgery? In elective cases, taking a few days to think about the procedure and get a second

opinion may be worth it in the long run. Furthermore, there is good evidence that people who have elective surgery do much better than those who undergo emergency surgery.

- Are you planning to repair or replace the valve? Risks increase when valves are repaired or replaced, so it is very important to know if this additional procedure is going to be performed and, if so, what the repercussions may be.
- What is the risk of death thirty days after surgery? What about ninety days or a year after? Are you worried about any specific complications in her case? How long will she stay in the hospital?
- Can you or your nurse show us the Society of Thoracic Surgeons calculator so we better understand the risks? A very good risk calculator from the Society of Thoracic Surgeons predicts the risk during CABG based on the person's age, sex, and medical history. People should expect the surgeon's nurse or nurse practitioner to review specific risks of CABG based on their individual profile. It is critical to consider the risks before opting for CABG.[1]
- Will you perform the surgery on or off a heart-lung machine? Ask the surgeon whether he plans to use a heart-lung machine, or pump, to take over the heart's function during the surgery. People who undergo "off-pump" surgery are at decreased risk for infection and heart rhythm issues after surgery. However, off-pump CABG poses a higher risk of anesthesia complications, kidney failure, heart attack, and stroke after surgery. The cardiologist or surgeon is the best judge of whether on or off pump is a good option, but off-pump surgeries should be performed only by surgeons with experience with them.

How Do We Prepare for CABG?

- Ensure that the person stops eating and drinking at midnight before the surgery.
- Remind the person to shower with soap or a special cleanser the night before and the morning of the surgery.
- Take all medicine bottles to the surgery.
- Ask the doctor whether any medicines need to be stopped before the procedure and, if so, when the person should take the last doses.
- Get all blood tests, ultrasounds, or lung function tests the surgeon or cardiologist orders.
- If the person has a pacemaker or defibrillator, tell the cardiologist or surgeon.

- Ensure that the person quits smoking as soon as she receives a diagnosis of coronary artery disease. If both the person and caregiver smoke, it is a good idea to quit together.

What Happens During CABG?

When you arrive at the hospital, you or the person are asked to complete paperwork to register for the surgery. Then the person is taken to a patient room, where these preparations are made:

- The person changes into a patient gown and removes any dentures or jewelry. A nurse checks the blood pressure, pulse, and temperature and places an intravenous (IV) line into the arm to draw blood for testing.
- The person signs a consent form giving the surgeon permission to perform the procedure and agreeing to the use of blood products in an emergency. The surgeon may review the risks and benefits of the procedure again.
- The anesthesiologist arrives and asks about any previous surgeries, general health, and any experience with anesthesia in the past. After the risks are explained, the person signs another consent form for the anesthesia. Other staff members helping the surgeon during the procedure arrive and introduce themselves. They may ask basic questions about health and medicines.
- The person empties her bladder and bowels and is taken to the operating room. Family members are asked to wait in the family area.

In the operating room, the person lies on her back on an operating table, and instruments to measure her heart rate, blood pressure, and oxygen levels are attached.

The person is given an IV anesthetic for sedation. Once the person is asleep, the anesthesiologist puts a breathing tube into her throat and connects it to a ventilator, which breathes for the person during the surgery. A catheter is placed in the bladder. The skin on the chest is cleaned with an antiseptic solution, and a sterile drape is placed over the rest of the body.

When this is done, the surgeon starts the surgery. He makes incisions in the chest, and an assistant does the same in the leg if leg veins are to be used for the bypass. The surgeon cuts the breastbone and spreads the ribs for a good view of the heart. The person is placed on a heart-lung machine if on-pump surgery is to be performed.

The surgeon performs the bypass surgery, grafting the arteries or veins onto the blocked coronary arteries. After the necessary bypass(es), the blood flow is checked.

The heart-lung machine is disconnected, and the heart returns to functioning as before.

Temporary metal wires are placed on the heart muscle, which function as a temporary pacemaker for the first two or three days after surgery.

The breastbone is reconnected with metal wires, and tubes are placed in the chest to drain blood and fluid from around the heart. The tissue under the skin and the skin itself is stitched, and a dressing is placed.

The person is transported to the recovery room and then to the intensive care unit (ICU), where blood pressure, heart rate, oxygenation, and electrocardiogram are continuously monitored.

Around this time, the anesthesia starts wearing off, and the person starts breathing on her own. The breathing machine is adjusted to allow the person to do so. The tube in her throat is removed once she is deemed strong enough to breathe completely on her own, which is usually the same day as the surgery but sometimes the next day.

Once the person is breathing on her own, she is encouraged to take deep breaths and cough every couple of hours. Someone shows her how to hug a pillow tightly to her chest while coughing to help ease the discomfort this causes. You should learn this technique to help the person follow it at home.

The surgeon places some tubes that come out of the chest. These tubes are removed on day two or three after the surgery.

If the person experiences pain, tell a staff member, who may give medicine, if appropriate.

The person may receive IV medicines to regulate her blood pressure and heart rate, but they will be slowly withdrawn during recovery. The person may start eating and drinking gradually once she can handle solids and liquids again.

Once the person does not need constant care and continuous monitoring, she is moved to another unit to recover further. Initially, she is asked to start walking with assistance and then by herself, with a staff member by her side. Cardiac rehabilitation starts before hospital release.

The physical therapist recommends exercises and their duration and intensity for at home. The person starts eating a heart-healthy diet. The temporary pacemaker wire is removed once deemed unnecessary, usually on day three or four.

Once the person can get out of bed and do some daily activities, she is released from the hospital.

You and the person need to understand the verbal and written instructions given at hospital release because it is important to understand:

- how to take care of the surgery site (e.g., dressing, cleaning);
- which medicines to take at home, including the dose, frequency, and use of each;
- if any previous medicines should be stopped and why;
- the dates and times of follow-up appointments with the surgeon and cardiologist;
- which activities to do and which to avoid;
- lifting restrictions and how long to follow them;
- whether the person can shower, details of any precautions, and the duration of these precautions and restrictions; and
- when the person should start cardiac rehabilitation and who will arrange it.

What Happens at Home After CABG?

The person should have someone drive her home from the hospital and have a caregiver at home for the first two to four weeks of recovery. You act as a nurse, coach, and assistant during this time.

Some of these symptoms may occur for as long as six weeks after CABG:

- pain in the chest around the incision,
- poor appetite,
- mood swings and "the blues,"
- momentary dizziness when getting up rapidly,
- swelling in the leg from where the vein was taken,
- itching and "pins and needles" sensation around the incision sites,
- constipation,
- feeling off or "fuzzy-headed," and
- poor energy level and fatigue.

The person should shower every day and wash the incision site gently with soap and water, taking care not to scrub the incision. Any white strips near the incision will fall off in a couple of weeks. If not, gently peel them off. The person should avoid using creams, lotions, and powders on the wound unless prescribed by the surgeon or cardiologist. For the first twelve weeks, the person should avoid hot tubs, baths, and swimming in lakes or oceans.

Poor appetite is common after surgery. The person may be constipated in the first two weeks. Fruit juice, fruits, and other high-fiber foods should help relieve constipation. A lifelong heart-healthy diet is recommended. It is important to remember that a poor diet, which led to blockages in the coronary arteries, can do the same thing after CABG. Refer to chapter 6 for further instructions.

Start activities gradually at home. Encourage the person to do the activities she did in the hospital before release, and gradually build on them over time to return to her normal activity level. Walking slowly and climbing stairs are good starting points. Avoid the outdoors if it is too cold or hot. The person should stop exercising if you notice that she has shortness of breath, dizziness, or chest pain. If these symptoms do not go away with rest, contact the doctor.

Talk to the cardiologist about a formal cardiac rehabilitation program. This program, under professional supervision, is the quickest way to return to regular activities and exercise. Refer to chapter 6 for information on home exercise after a cardiac rehabilitation program.

The person should avoid activities that pull on the incision (e.g., rowing, weight lifting, swimming, golfing). Discourage the person from using her arms to lift herself from a chair. Help her rise from a chair in the early recovery period.

Discourage pushing or pulling objects heavier than ten pounds. The person should avoid activities that require the arms to be above the shoulders for longer than fifteen minutes for six weeks. The person will be given a small pillow to hold over her chest when she coughs or takes deep breaths. Encourage regular use of this pillow.

You should be the designated driver for six weeks while the person cannot drive.

If there is an incision on the leg, encourage the person to keep her leg raised while sitting. Encourage her to wear elastic TED hose on the leg until she is more active. Encourage movement every couple of hours.

After the first three weeks, you may delegate light household chores to the person.

The person should avoid travel for the first six weeks.

The person should avoid sex for the first six weeks. She may resume sex after six weeks, keeping wound care restrictions in mind.

Although depression and "the blues" after CABG may cause a lack of interest in sex, most people recover from these mood changes within three months. Because most caregivers are the spouse, they can help follow these instructions.

Encourage the person to re-engage with hobbies and social activities.

Most people can return to a desk job in four weeks. People who do light physical work may return after about eight weeks, after receiving permission from their doctor.

Encourage the person to get eight hours of sleep a night. Discourage naps during the day and caffeine, soda, and caffeinated tea in the evening. Discourage screen time one hour before bed.[2]

Use Tylenol or Extra Strength Tylenol for pain. If it does not relieve the pain, contact the surgeon's office.

When Should I Call the Doctor's Office?

Watch for the following situations, and seek medical advice immediately if they arise:

- a fever of 100.4 degrees Fahrenheit (38 degrees Celsius) or higher;
- redness, swelling, bleeding, or other drainage from any incision site;
- ongoing cough a week after surgery or coughing up blood or green sputum;
- an increase in pain around any incision site;
- difficulty breathing at rest;
- fluttering in the chest or rapid heartbeat;
- numbness in the arms or legs;
- ongoing nausea or vomiting;
- chest pain, shortness of breath, or arm pain with activity that does not go away with rest;
- dizziness or lightheadedness at rest; or
- the breastbone feels like it shifts, pops, or cracks with movement.

What Long-Term Changes Are Recommended After Recovery From CABG?

Blockages in the coronary arteries for which CABG is performed can build up again over time. Avoiding the rebuilding of blockages should be the number one health priority. The person should switch to a heart-healthy diet, quit smoking, get regular exercise, and manage stress. You have a critical role in cultivating and implementing these lifelong habits.

Angioplasty

Angioplasty is a procedure to open a blocked coronary artery and restore normal blood flow to the heart muscle.

Balloon Angioplasty

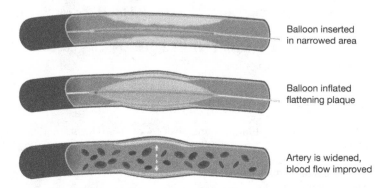

Balloon inserted in narrowed area

Balloon inflated flattening plaque

Artery is widened, blood flow improved

Figure 5.8. Angioplasty is a procedure to open a blocked coronary artery and restore normal blood flow to the heart muscle. © *iStock/ Getty Images Plus/solar22*

The doctor accesses the artery in the arm or groin. Through it, he threads a small, long, flexible plastic tube called a catheter into the coronary artery. Using the catheter as a channel, he passes another thinner, balloon-tipped catheter through the catheter deep inside the coronary artery. He inflates the balloon within the blockage, pushing away the plaque that is blocking the blood flow. The passage is thus widened, and blood flow in the coronary artery is restored.

Angioplasty is often combined with the placement of a small wire mesh tube called a stent to open the artery and decrease the chance of it narrowing again.

When Is Angioplasty Performed?

Angioplasty is done when blockages in one or more coronary arteries are detected. On occasion, it is done in an emergency when the person is having a life-threatening heart attack due to 100 percent blockage of a coronary artery.

Most often, an angioplasty is done if a person is found to have a more than 70 percent blockage in a coronary artery during a scheduled cardiac catheterization. Combined with medicine, angioplasty relieves symptoms related to coronary artery disease.

How Does the Person Prepare for the Procedure?

The preparation for angioplasty is the same as that for cardiac catheterization. The doctor's office gives written instructions about the procedure and may call with further instructions. Write down the information and follow it closely. The general guidelines to preparing for an angioplasty are:

- Do not eat or drink anything from midnight until after the procedure.
- Bring all medicine bottles to the procedure.
- People with diabetes need to understand the specific advice about taking their diabetes pills or insulin injection.
- People taking blood thinners (warfarin, Coumadin, Jantoven, Eliquis, Pradaxa, or Xarelto) need to understand the directions about stopping these medicines.

What Happens When the Person Arrives at the Hospital for the Procedure?

On arrival at the hospital, you or the person completes the paperwork and checks in for the procedure. Then you and the person are brought into a patient room in the catheterization lab area, where the person is prepared for the procedure:

- The person changes into a hospital gown and removes any dentures or jewelry.
- A nurse checks the person's blood pressure, pulse, and temperature.
- A nurse inserts an intravenous (IV) line and draws blood for testing.
- A nurse shaves the groin or arm where the catheter will be inserted.
- You or the person signs a consent form to give the doctor permission to perform the procedure and give blood products in an emergency, if needed. The doctor may review the risks and benefits of the procedure again, verify general health information, verify any previous problems the person has had with medicine or anesthesia, and answer any questions.
- The person may want to use the restroom before being taken to the procedure room while the family members go to the waiting area.

What Happens During the Procedure?

The person is taken to the catheterization lab for the procedure, where she lies on a special table and is given medicines through the IV to stay relaxed and pain-free. She will likely be semi-awake during the procedure.

Staff place soft, sticky patches called electrodes on her chest, arms, and legs for an electrocardiogram. A staff member prepares the site of cardiac catheterization and covers the person in a sterile drape.

The doctor injects local anesthesia at the site of the catheterization. Once the area is numb, he uses a needle to access the artery and inserts a plastic tube called a sheath. He passes the catheter through the sheath into the coronary artery.

Once the catheter is in position, he injects dye and takes X-ray pictures of the coronary arteries. He takes multiple pictures by repositioning the X-ray machine around the person's body to see the arteries from many angles. The person may be asked to take a deep breath or hold her breath during parts of the procedure.

If a blockage is detected, the doctor tells the person the findings and performs the angioplasty.

The previously inserted catheter is replaced with another, stiffer catheter. Using this catheter as a channel, he passes a thinner, balloon-tipped catheter into the blocked coronary artery. The balloon at the end of the catheter is inflated (opened) and then deflated. The plaque that created the blockage is pushed to the wall of the artery, widening the artery and restoring blood flow.

The doctor removes the balloon-tipped catheter. If a stent is needed, the doctor places it in the recently opened coronary artery. The stent locks in place inside the artery and keeps it open. Sometimes more than one stent is required. The stent is left inside the artery, and all catheters are removed. The procedure is complete.

The doctor may tell you and the person the results of the procedure.

What Happens After the Procedure?

The staff removes the sterile drape and takes the person to the recovery room, possibly the same room where she prepared for the procedure. They remove the plastic sheath from the groin or arm and apply pressure to the site to prevent bleeding. If the insertion site was the groin, the person lies flat for several hours.

She can eat and drink after the procedure. The person may be released the same day or the next day, depending on the situation. Before release, the person receives detailed instructions on any new medicines. She should make an appointment for a follow-up visit with the doctor.

How Do I Care for the Person After the Procedure?

Ensure that the person drinks eight to ten glasses of water in the twenty-four hours after the procedure. The next morning, wet the small bandage at the groin or arm site and remove it. Gently wash the site with soap and water once a day for the next five days. Keep the area dry the rest of the time. Do not use creams or lotions at the site. For the first week, the person should avoid wearing tight clothes and getting into a hot tub, pool, or lake.

Watch for bruising around the site, which is normal. It is not unusual to have a small lump the size of a quarter. However, if you notice that the lump is growing or painful, contact the doctor.

The person, who may feel tired the day after the procedure, should rest and take walks around the house for the first two days. The person should avoid strenuous activities such as running and golfing for a week and climb any stairs slowly. After the first week, the person can gradually increase daily activities.

Do not put pressure on the groin or arm site. If the groin was used, the person should not strain during bowel movements for a week after the procedure. If she has constipation, she can use laxatives during this time. The person should not lift more than ten pounds and avoid pushing or pulling anything heavy for a week.

Most people are able to resume driving in one or two days, a desk job in two or three days, and sex in a week.

Call the doctor if you notice:

- bleeding or swelling at the site of the procedure (arm or leg);
- pain, redness, fever, drainage, or swelling at the site of the procedure;
- lightheadedness or dizziness; or
- chest pain or shortness of breath.

How Are the Results Reported?

The result is reported as a percentage of blockage in different coronary arteries (e.g., 40 percent stenosis in the right coronary artery and 30 percent blockage in the left main artery). It will also mention which artery was opened up and the amount of narrowing before and after the angioplasty. The angioplasty report card that the person will be given mentions which artery was opened and the size of the stent used and may be needed later. The person should either carry this card or a picture of it on his or her phone.

How Do I Take Care of the Person's Health?

Once the person has undergone angioplasty, she should follow this advice for all people:

- Exercise regularly.
- Discuss dietary recommendations with the doctor or dietitian.
- Consider a whole, plant-based diet.
- Maintain weight in the normal range.
- If the person has diabetes, try to maintain strict control of blood sugar.
- Keep blood pressure at less than 120/80 mm Hg.
- Quit smoking.
- Use alcohol strictly in moderation.
- Understand prescribed medicines and their uses.
- Recognize heart disease–related symptoms.

What Are the Risks of Angioplasty?

As with all invasive procedures, angioplasty carries risks. A person needs to carefully consider these potential complications before undergoing angioplasty:

- heart attack due to clot formation within the stent;
- damage to the blood vessel where the catheter was inserted;
- heart attack due to sudden closure of the coronary artery;
- tears in the lining of the coronary artery;
- risk of urgent bypass surgery due to angioplasty-related complications;
- reblocking of the coronary artery where angioplasty was done (without stent placement, this happens in 30 percent of people; with a stent, this happens in 10 percent to 15 percent of people);
- bleeding at the site where the tiny tube was inserted;
- damage to the kidneys from use of the dye;
- stroke; or
- death.

In addition to these major complications, these other complications may occur:

- bruising or blood accumulation in the arm or groin,
- damage to the artery of the arm or groin (pseudoaneurysm),
- irregular heart rhythms (arrhythmias), or
- allergic reaction to the IV dye.

What Questions Should We Ask the Cardiologist Before Having an Angioplasty?

All decisions about treatment should be based on the individual condition in consultation with the doctor. To make a well-informed decision, you or the person should ask the cardiologist these questions:

- Which arteries are blocked?
- What is the percentage of the blockage?
- Is this an elective or emergency angioplasty?
- Can we try medicine to address the symptoms first?
- Will the person live longer if they have the angioplasty?
- What are the risks of the procedure?
- Is the person in the high-risk category?
- Which symptoms will improve after angioplasty?
- Will the person need blood thinners after the angioplasty? Will she tolerate them?

Is It Better to Open a Blocked Coronary Artery with Angioplasty Rather Than with Medicine?

Angioplasty can be life-saving during a life-threatening heart attack. Intuitively, it makes sense that opening blocked arteries is better for the person. However, people who have angioplasty in a non-heart-attack situation have not been shown to live longer than those who do not.

Angioplasty helps relieve chest pain and shortness of breath when used along with heart medicines. It does not lower the risk of a heart attack in the future and, in fact, may even increase the short-term risk of a heart attack.

Ablation

What Is Ablation?

Ablation is an invasive procedure to eliminate heart rhythm problems. The doctor gets access into the vein in the groin and threads small, thin, flexible tubes called catheters into different parts of the heart. She then maps the heart to find the tissue causing the problem and cauterizes (burns) this tissue with a catheter to get rid of the heart rhythm problem.

When Is Ablation Recommended?

The doctor recommends ablation for supraventricular tachycardia if it lasts a long time and causes palpitations, lightheadedness, dizziness, or excessive fatigue. Medicines can be used instead of ablation.

A doctor recommends an ablation for atrial fibrillation if it causes palpitations, shortness of breath, lightheadedness, or dizziness. Ablation is not recommended if the person does not have these symptoms. If the person's only symptom is fatigue, the doctor must verify that it is caused by atrial fibrillation before performing ablation. In most cases, medicines are used before ablation and can be equally effective. However, if the person wants to avoid medicines, ablation may be done instead.

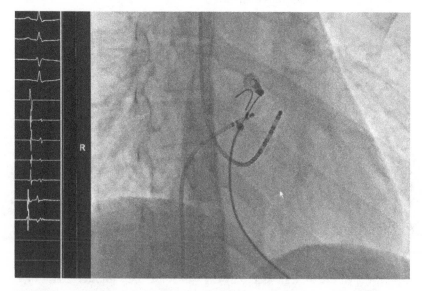

Figure 5.9. Ablation, an invasive procedure to cure heart rhythm problems. © iStock/Getty Images Plus/zilli

What Questions Should We Ask If the Doctor Recommends Ablation?

- Which symptoms are we trying to address with ablation?
- What is the risk of long-term complications from the arrhythmia?
- Could another condition be causing these symptoms?
- What are the specific risks from the procedure?
- Does the person have risk factors for complications?
- Can the person try medical treatment and lifestyle changes before ablation?
- What medicines can be safely stopped after ablation?

What Are the Risks of the Procedure?

Like all invasive procedures, ablation has its risks, such as:

- puncture of the heart wall, causing blood to seep out of the heart (tamponade);
- stroke;
- damage to the coronary artery;
- damage to the nerve supplying the diaphragm, causing shortness of breath;
- an abnormal and potentially fatal connection between the heart and the esophagus (food pipe);
- blood clots to the lungs;
- kidney damage;
- infection; or
- death.

Other complications can also occur, such as:

- bruising or blood accumulation in the groin,
- damage to the groin vein (pseudoaneurysm), or
- irregular heart rhythms (arrhythmias).

How Should I Prepare the Person for the Procedure?

The doctor's office will call before the procedure to give instructions. You should write down these instructions. The general guidelines in preparation for an ablation procedure are:

- The person should not eat or drink anything after midnight before the procedure.

- Take all medicine bottles to the procedure.
- People with diabetes may need to stop or alter their dose of diabetes pills and/or insulin injections.
- People who take beta blockers (e.g., metoprolol, atenolol), calcium channel blockers (e.g., diltiazem, verapamil), or another rhythm-related medicine will receive instructions for stopping or continuing them before the procedure.
- People who take blood thinners (warfarin, Coumadin, Jantoven, Eliquis, Pradaxa, or Xarelto) need to understand the doctor's directions for stopping these medicines. If no guidance is given, ask for it.
- In some cases, the doctor may request an echocardiogram or computed tomographic (CT) scan before the procedure. Ensure that it is completed prior to the procedure.

What Happens at the Hospital Before the Procedure?

You or the person complete paperwork and check in for the ablation. The person is taken to a room in the electrophysiology lab area, where these steps are taken to prepare for the procedure:

- changing into a patient gown and removing any dentures or jewelry;
- checking the person's blood pressure, pulse, and temperature;
- inserting an intravenous (IV) line into the person's arm and drawing blood for testing;
- shaving the person's groin and chest;
- signing the consent form to give the doctor permission to perform the procedure and use blood products, if needed, during an emergency (the doctor may review the risks and benefits of the procedure and answer any questions);
- signing the consent form to give the anesthesiologist permission to use sedatives (if the person has had trouble with anesthesia in the past, advise the anesthesiologist or staff);
- verifying information about the person's general health;
- verifying any previous problems the person had with medicines; and
- using the restroom to empty the bladder or bowel before the procedure.

What Happens During the Procedure?

The person is transferred to the electrophysiology lab for the procedure. He lies on a special table and is given IV medicine to keep him relaxed and pain-free. He will be semi-awake or asleep for the procedure.

Staff place multiple soft, sticky patches on the person's chest, arms, and legs to monitor the electrocardiogram and perform arrhythmia mapping. If the person is to be sedated completely, the anesthesiologist gives him medicine and places a breathing tube, if needed. In many cases, the person is made sleepy and pain free but not totally asleep. The staff covers the person in a sterile drape.

The doctor injects local anesthesia. Once the area is numb, she inserts a needle into the vein in one or both groins and places plastic tubes called sheaths. She passes multiple catheters through the sheaths into different parts of the heart. Once the catheters are placed, the doctor maps the arrhythmia and then cauterizes or freezes the heart tissue causing the rhythm problem. This procedure may take minutes to hours.

The doctor removes the catheter, the sedation is stopped, and the person wakes. The doctor informs the family and caregivers whether the procedure was successful and if there were any complications.

What Happens After the Procedure?

The sterile drape is removed, and the person is taken to the recovery room, which may be the same room where he prepared for the procedure. The plastic sheath in the groin or chest is removed, and a staff member applies pressure to the insertion sites. The person must lay flat for several hours. He can eat and drink once he is fully awake.

The time of hospital release depends on the treatment plan, which is based on the results of the procedure. The doctor or a team member gives specific instructions to be followed at home. You should understand instructions about:

- activity restrictions;
- shower and bathing restrictions;
- driving restrictions;
- changes in medicine, if any;

- care of the wound site and dressing;
- pain management;
- return to work;
- follow-up appointment with the doctor; and
- situations in which the doctor's office should be contacted.

How Do I Care for the Person After the Procedure?

Before leaving the hospital, get an updated list of medicines to be used. Ensure that you understand any new medicine to start and any previous medicines to be stopped. Make a follow-up appointment for the person.

The person should drink eight to ten glasses of water during the twenty-four hours after the procedure.

The person will have a small bandage on his groin. The next morning, wet the bandage and remove it. Wash this area gently with soap and water once a day for the next five days. Keep the area dry the rest of the time, and do not use creams or lotions. The person should avoid wearing tight clothes for the first week and getting into a hot tub, pool, or lake for seven days.

The person may have bruising or a quarter-sized lump around the site, which is normal. However, if the lump increases or is painful, contact the doctor.

The person may feel tired the day after the procedure and should rest and walk around the house for the first two days. He should avoid strenuous activities such as running and golfing for a week. After the first week, he can gradually be more active.

Do not put pressure on the groin where the procedure was done. The person should not strain during bowel movements for the first week. He should avoid lifting more than ten pounds or pushing or pulling anything heavy during this time.

Most people can resume driving in one or two days, a desk job in two or three days, and sex in a week.

When Should I Call the Doctor's Office?

Watch for the following situations, and seek medical advice immediately in case of:

- fever of 100.4 degrees Fahrenheit (38 degrees Celsius) or higher;
- swelling, bleeding, or other drainage from the wound site;
- ongoing cough a week after surgery or coughing up blood;

- difficulty breathing at rest;
- slurred speech, headaches, or weakness in the arms or legs;
- palpitations or fluttering in the chest;
- rapid heartbeat;
- numbness in the arms or legs;
- chest pain, shortness of breath, or arm pain with activity that does not go away with rest; and
- dizziness or lightheadedness at rest.

Pacemakers

What Is the Normal Electrical System of the Heart?

The heart's own electrical system generates the electricity it needs. The heart's spark plug, the sinoatrial (SA) node in the right upper chamber, starts a normal heartbeat. From here, the electrical activity spreads to the two upper chambers. The electricity then conducts to the atrioventricular (AV) junction, located between the upper and lower chambers. After a minor delay, the electricity spreads to the lower chamber.

Contraction of the heart chambers follows the spread of electricity in the same pattern. In a normal heart, the upper chambers get the electrical signal and then contract. After a brief delay, the lower chamber receives electrical impulses and contracts in a rhythmic, coordinated manner.

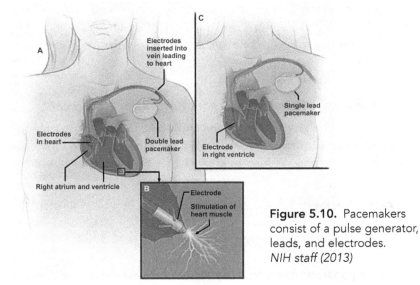

Figure 5.10. Pacemakers consist of a pulse generator, leads, and electrodes. *NIH staff (2013)*

Our brain and body require 50 to 100 beats a minute to be properly supplied with oxygenated blood. Fewer than the required beats are produced when one of the following things occurs:

- The SA node slows and produces an inadequate number of heart beats.
- The AV junction between the upper and lower chambers is damaged. Therefore, it is not able to send each beat from the upper chamber to the lower chamber.

When Is a Pacemaker Needed?

The doctor may recommend a pacemaker if the person has:

- fatigue, lightheadedness, or fainting from a low heart rate;
- inability to exercise because the heart rate does not increase enough during exercise; or
- damage to the electrical system of the heart during heart valve surgery.

What Is a Pacemaker? How Does It Work?

A permanent (artificial) pacemaker has two parts:

- A pulse generator: A small metal container with a battery and electrical circuitry. It goes under the skin next to the left or right shoulder and controls the electrical activity of the heart. Sometimes it is called a pacemaker or battery.
- Leads and electrodes: Wires that travel from the pulse generator to the heart. They connect the heart to the electrical circuitry in the pulse generator.

How Should the Person Prepare for Pacemaker Placement?

The doctor's office gives written instructions about the procedure and may call with further instructions. Write down the information, and follow it closely. The general guidelines to preparing for the pacemaker placement procedure are:

- Ensure that the person stops eating and drinking by midnight before the surgery.
- Remind the person to shower with soap or a special cleanser the night before.
- Get all presurgery blood tests ordered by the doctor.

- Ask the doctor if medicines such as blood thinners (e.g., warfarin) need to be stopped before the procedure and, if so, when the person should take the last dose. If the person has diabetes, ask whether she should take her diabetes pills or insulin injection the morning of surgery.
- Take all medicines along to the surgery.

What Happens at the Hospital Before the Procedure?

When you arrive at the hospital, you or the person complete the paperwork to register for the procedure. Then the person is taken to a patient room, where these preparations are made:

- person changing into a gown;
- removing any dentures or jewelry;
- checking blood pressure, pulse, and temperature;
- placing an intravenous (IV) line in the arm to draw blood for testing;
- shaving and cleaning the chest; and
- signing the consent form to give permission to perform the surgery and blood transfusion, if needed.

Staff members helping the cardiologist introduce themselves and ask questions about the person's health, previous surgeries, allergies, and any experiences with anesthesia.

The person uses the restroom and is taken to the operating room. Family members wait in the family area.

What Happens During the Procedure?

The person is taken to a lab, where she lies on a special table, and instruments to measure her heart rate, blood pressure, and oxygen levels are attached. She is given medicines through the IV. She may be semi-awake during the procedure.

Staff place soft, sticky patches called electrodes on her chest, arms, and legs for an electrocardiogram. A staff member prepares the site of pacemaker placement and covers the person in a sterile drape.

The doctor injects local anesthesia at the site of the pacemaker. Once the area is numb, the doctor makes an incision and uses a needle to access the vein. He places a plastic sheath in the vein near the collarbone.

He passes the lead or leads into the heart through the sheath and monitors the position of the lead with an X-ray machine. Once the leads are well placed in the heart, the doctor tests the leads. If the lead passes the test, it is tied to the muscles near the collarbone. He creates a space for the pacemaker, washes the space with an antibiotic solution, connects the pacemaker generator to the lead, and places it in the space. The doctor closes the incision with sutures and applies adhesive strips, glue, or staples and a sterile dressing.

The sterile drape is removed. The blood pressure and oxygen monitoring devices are disconnected, and team members transfer the person to the recovery area.

After the Procedure

In the recovery area, the person's electrocardiogram, blood pressure, and oxygenation are monitored. Once the person is awake, she can eat and drink. At this time, family members are allowed to visit and stay with the person and should report any unusual symptoms (e.g., chest pain, breathing difficulty) to the nurse.

After a rest period, the person may get out of bed with assistance and, later, independently. Once her blood pressure, pulse, and breathing are stable, the person is discharged to home or transferred to a hospital room. Some doctors prefer to keep the person for a one-night stay in the hospital. In such cases, the next morning, the pacemaker is checked, and a chest X-ray is done. If all tests are normal, the person is released to home.

The doctor or a team member give specific instructions to be followed at home.

You should understand instructions about:

- activity restrictions;
- driving restrictions;
- restrictions on moving the arm;
- restrictions on lifting the arm;
- changes in medicine, if any;
- care of the wound site and dressing;
- shower and bathing restrictions;
- pain management;
- return to work;
- follow-up appointment with the doctor;
- follow-up appointment at the pacemaker clinic, where the pacemaker is checked; and
- situations in which the doctor's office should be contacted.

A card that gives details about the pacemaker and a monitoring device that transmits information from the pacemaker to the doctor's office are provided. Place the monitoring device by the person's bed at home. If this is not provided before release from the hospital, ask for it.

At Home

You may need to take time off of work to care for the person over the next few days.

The person should rest when tired but gradually increase her activity level. The person should not drive for four to six weeks. You should coordinate plans to be able to drive to doctor's appointments.

Lifting is restricted to ten pounds for two to four weeks. The person should not raise the arm on the side of the pacemaker above the shoulder for the first week. She should keep the arm active otherwise; you should remind the person about this. The person needs help from you to follow these restrictions (e.g., to reach objects placed high up, comb hair, get up from bed).

While sleeping, the person may accidentally raise her arm to support her head. You should remind the person of the arm restrictions and suggest that she use an arm sling at night to avoid accidentally raising the arm.

Encourage the person to start activities gradually at home. Walking slowly and climbing stairs are good starting points that she can gradually build on over time. Avoid the outdoors if it is too cold or hot. Vigorous exercise, swimming, golfing, and pushing a lawn mower should be avoided for six weeks. The person can go back to work one or two weeks after surgery. She should avoid sex for the first four weeks.

Follow the wound care instructions. Ensure that the wound does not get wet for seven days by avoiding baths and hot tubs. The person can take sponge baths during this time. After seven days, the doctor may let her take a shower. Any white strips at the surgical site will fall off on their own. Do not apply lotion, powder, or ointment to the surgical site.

The wound will be sore for about two weeks. Prescription painkillers should be used sparingly. Mild bruising and swelling of the surgical site will resolve over four weeks.

Remind the person to drink eight to ten glasses of water starting the day after the procedure. Help the person get back to her routine diet.

If you notice any of the following, notify the doctor's office immediately:

- fever and/or chills;
- increased pain, redness, swelling, bleeding, or other drainage from the site;

- chest pain or pressure;
- excessive sweating, dizziness, or lightheadedness; or
- palpitations.

How Do I Care for the Pacemaker for the Next Few Years?

- Ensure that the monitoring device is connected and placed next to the person's bed.
- Keep regular appointments with the pacemaker clinic.
- Report any redness, swelling, bleeding, or drainage at the site of the wound.
- Ensure that the person carries the pacemaker ID card, which includes the name and model number of the pacemaker. The person should wear a medical alert bracelet indicating that she has a pacemaker.
- At the airport, tell security about the pacemaker so they can ensure that the person can safely go through the metal detectors.
- If a doctor prescribes magnetic resonance imaging (MRI), tell him about the pacemaker. Some pacemakers are safe to go through MRI, while others are not.
- Before any surgery, tell the surgeon about the pacemaker.
- Remind the person to avoid activities that can injure the site of the pacemaker (e.g., playing softball).
- The person can use devices like microwave ovens, televisions, remote controls, radios, toasters, electric blankets, electric shavers, electric drills, and other household electrical items. If the person plans to use a new type of electrical equipment, clear it with the pacemaker clinic first.
- The person can use cell phones but should not put the cell phone in the pocket next to the pacemaker.
- Ensure that the person stands more than two feet away from welding equipment, high-voltage transformers, and motor-generator systems at all times. Large motors may create a magnetic field that could affect the pacemaker. If the person is repairing a car, boat, RV, or other vehicle, she should turn off the large motor of the vehicle.
- The person should avoid large magnetic fields such as those from power generation sites, automobile junkyards, and some manufacturing units. Remind the person to avoid high-voltage or radar machinery, such as radio or television transmitters, electric arc welders, high-tension wires, radar installations, and smelting furnaces.

Implantable Cardioverter Defibrillators

The heart's electrical system generates the electricity required for heartbeats. The heart's spark plug, the sinoatrial node in the right upper chamber, starts a normal heartbeat. From there, the electrical activity spreads to the two upper chambers and then to the atrioventricular junction, a bridge between the upper and lower chambers. After a minor delay, the electricity spreads to the lower chamber.

Contraction of the heart chambers follows the spread of electricity in the same pattern. In a normal heart, the upper chambers get the electrical signal and then contract. After a brief delay, the lower chamber receives electrical impulses and contracts in a rhythmic, coordinated manner. Our hearts beat in this way 50 to 100 beats a minute.

Occasionally, the normal heart rhythm gets disrupted, and people have an abnormal rhythm. Most abnormal rhythms are harmless. However, people with advanced heart disease can have a heart rhythm from the lower chambers (ventricles) called ventricular tachycardia/ventricular fibrillation (VT/VF), which disrupts normal blood flow to the body and quickly becomes life threatening. People may have chest pain, shortness of breath, palpitations, or dizziness or may simply collapse within seconds, requiring immediate medical attention.

What Should I Do if the Person Has VT/VF?

VT/VF is a life-threatening emergency. If the person collapses, you must:

- Call 911.
- Check for a pulse.
- If there is no pulse, begin cardiopulmonary resuscitation (CPR). Many caregivers learn how to perform CPR.
- If a portable automated external defibrillator (AED) is available, use it immediately if a second person is available to do so without interrupting CPR. AEDs are often available in public places such as a shopping mall, police car, sports stadium, and restaurant. Most AEDs come with built-in instructions and will only deliver a shock when needed.

When the emergency services arrive, they will take over and transfer the person to the nearest emergency department.

Who Gets VT/VF?

VT/VF can occur within the first hours or days after a heart attack. People with a weak heart, or cardiomyopathy, can also have these life-threatening arrhythmias. People with rare genetic conditions (e.g., Brugada syndrome, long QT syndrome, hypertrophic cardiomyopathy) can also have VT/VF.

What Is an ICD?

An ICD has two parts:

- A pulse generator, a small metal container the size of a pocket watch with a battery and electrical circuitry: It goes under the skin next to the left shoulder. It receives information from the heart via the leads and provides electrical shocks if the person has VT/VF.
- Leads or wires that connect the pulse generator to the heart.

Who Needs an ICD?

People who have been revived from VT/VF are at risk for another such incident. They are ideal candidates for an ICD. Others who may require an ICD preemptively are people with:

- ejection fraction, a measure of the heart's pumping strength, of less than 35 percent (normal, 55 percent to 70 percent) despite use of medicines to improve it, or
- rare genetic diseases such as long QT syndrome, Brugada syndrome, hypertrophic cardiomyopathy, or arrhythmogenic right ventricular dysplasia.

If the Person Has Advanced Heart Disease, Should an ICD Be Placed?

ICD prevents the person from dying of fatal VT/VF. People of advanced age and those with multiple medical conditions or dementia may not wish to be revived. In such cases, the person and family should discuss the need for an ICD with the doctor. It is important to understand how the ICD can and cannot benefit the person. For example, if the person is eighty-five years old, has a poor quality of life due to multiple medical problems, and is comfortable with the idea of dying, a fatal VT/VF in the middle of the night is the ideal way to go. In that case, an ICD is not a good option. However, if the person enjoys a good quality of life and wants to be revived from VT/VF, an

ICD should be considered. You can discuss this with the person, family, and health care team before ICD implantation.

The person should understand that an ICD does not strengthen the heart. It shocks the heart out of VT/VF rhythm but does not improve the ejection fraction.

How Should the Person Prepare for ICD Placement?

The preparation for ICD placement is similar to that of the pacemaker (reviewed earlier in this chapter).

What Happens at the Hospital Before, During, and After the Procedure?

The surgical procedure and after care of the ICD is similar to that of the pacemaker (reviewed earlier in this chapter).

How Do I Take Care of the Person After ICD Placement?

The care at home immediately after and in the years to come is similar to that after pacemaker placement (reviewed earlier in this chapter).

What Should I Do If the ICD Shocks the Person?

If the person gets one ICD shock and then feels normal again, call the doctor's office. If she gets more than one shock or continues to feel lightheaded, faints, is short of breath, or has palpitations, call 911.

Left Ventricular Assist Devices

A left ventricular assist device (LVAD) is a pump that assists the pumping function of the heart. It takes blood from the heart and pushes it into the aorta and the rest of the body. The pump gets electricity from an outlet or battery attached to a cable.

An LVAD does not replace the heart but helps a weak heart. An LVAD is not a cure for heart failure but an adjunct to other treatments for heart failure. It is implanted during open heart surgery. Occasionally, both the right and the left side of the heart are weak, in which case a biventricular assist device (BiVAD) is placed instead of an LVAD. Different kinds of LVADs are available on the market.

All LVADs have four parts:

- A pump takes the blood from the heart into the aorta.
- The pump is connected to a cable called the driveline. This cable passes from the pump through the skin into the controller and supplies electricity to the pump. It also sends information from the controller to the pump, and vice versa.
- The controller is a small computer that sits outside the body and controls the pump.
- A power unit provides electricity to the pump. This consists of rechargeable batteries or a cord that plugs into an electrical outlet.

HeartMate 3, HeartMate 2, and HeartWare are different brands of LVADs approved by the US Food and Drug Administration.

When Will the Doctor Recommend an LVAD?

An LVAD is a treatment option for a certain group of people with weak heart function and congestive heart failure. Most people undergo multiple medical and surgical treatments to improve the function of their heart before being considered for LVAD. A caregiver willing to provide round-the-clock care for six months or longer is a necessary condition before the person is considered for LVAD.

Even among this select group of people, LVAD is not a good option for people with:

- poor kidney function,
- abnormal liver function,
- blood-clotting problems,
- advanced lung disease,
- high propensity for infection, or
- serious mental illness.

Some people receive an LVAD while awaiting heart transplantation. In these people, it helps improve the person's symptoms until they undergo heart transplantation. The LVAD is removed at the time of heart transplantation.

Another group of people receive an LVAD when they continue to have symptoms of heart failure after all other treatment options have been exhausted and heart transplantation is not an option. In these people, an LVAD improves the person's symptoms for the rest of their lives. Rarely, an

LVAD is placed until the person's own heart recovers, after which the LVAD is removed.

What Is My Role After the Person Receives an LVAD?

The person is considered for an LVAD if a caregiver is willing to help the person round the clock for the first six months after LVAD surgery. In many cases, it becomes a lifelong responsibility for you.

You learn to care for the LVAD in addition to helping the person with activities of daily living. You learn to manage the LVAD by changing the dressings on the LVAD cables, monitoring for infections, and managing the power supply. This is in addition to managing daily medicines, helping with activities of daily living, meeting daily dietary needs, transporting the person to and from clinic visits, and providing emotional support.

What Are the Benefits of an LVAD?

An LVAD boosts the pumping function of the heart and increases blood flow to the body. Increased blood flow to the brain, kidneys, and liver ensures proper functioning of these organs. It improves the person's strength and ability to participate in activities. People with an LVAD have fewer symptoms related to heart failure (e.g., shortness of breath, fatigue). Overall, an LVAD lengthens the life span of people with heart failure and offers better quality of life.

What Are the Risks of an LVAD?

People with a weak heart and congestive heart failure have weak immune systems; thus, there is an increased risk of infection with LVAD surgery. Other risks involve problems with bleeding and clotting. People with clotting problems may have a stroke. Another concern in people with an LVAD is the possibility of kidney failure.

Like any complex machine, LVADs can malfunction. Caregivers can help with early detection of these complications and work with the health care team to prevent and treat them.

How Does the Person Prepare for LVAD Surgery?

The health care team meets with the person, family, and caregiver multiple times to understand the disease and its impact on the person. The person's other medical conditions, mental health, family situation, and overall well-being are considered before LVAD surgery is offered and undertaken.

The team reviews the risks of LVAD surgery and the care of the person and the LVAD after surgery. The preoperative guidelines for LVAD surgery are similar to those of coronary artery bypass grafting (CABG, reviewed earlier in this chapter).

What Happens During LVAD Surgery?

The pre-surgical steps are similar to those of CABG surgery. The surgery is performed under general anesthesia and takes four to six hours.

The surgeon makes an incision in the chest and opens and splits the breastbone to reach the heart. She attaches the heart to a heart-lung bypass machine to provide blood to the body while she operates on the heart. Then she attaches the LVAD pump to the heart. A tube, or cannula, connects the pump to the aorta. A cable is connected to the pump and brought out through the skin in the abdomen before the incision is closed.

After the surgery, the person stays in the intensive care unit for a few days before moving to a regular hospital room. The person remains in the hospital after LVAD surgery for fourteen to twenty-one days.

Recovery from LVAD surgery is similar to that after CABG surgery (reviewed earlier in this chapter).

The LVAD person requires care of the wound site and the LVAD. During hospitalization, you are taught different aspects of LVAD care:

- You are taught to change dressings on the wound where the cable emerges from the abdomen. Dressing changes as advised by the team prevent infection. You have an opportunity to practice this under the supervision of the health care team before the person leaves the hospital.
- The LVAD monitor displays numbers indicating pump flow and speed, pulse index, and power. The person and caregiver are taught about these numbers and their importance during the hospital stay. They become familiar and comfortable with these numbers before leaving the hospital.
- You and the person learn how to switch between batteries and the power module as the power source. The nurse demonstrates it, and you have the opportunity to practice it multiple times during the hospital stay.
- An LVAD self-test should be done daily. The person and caregiver learn the steps for this test and how to interpret the information provided by an LVAD self-test. You are given information on critical situations in which you should contact the health care team.

Aftercare in People With an LVAD

After the person is released from the hospital, he will have appointments with the health care team once a week for the first several weeks. During these visits, the team will monitor the person's recovery and check the LVAD's functioning. You can clarify any concerns about home care of the person and LVAD.

After the surgery the person has several visits with a physical therapist, occupational therapist, home health nurse, and others to help him and you transition from the post-surgery period to daily life. In addition to watching for complications from the surgery or LVAD, this team helps the person incorporate healthy lifestyle changes (e.g., exercise, diet, stress management). The team is a great support for you and the person.

When Should I Contact the Team?

All guidelines discussed above about contacting the doctor's office for people apply to LVAD people. Also, you should contact the health care team if any of the following events occur:

- increased pump pulse pressure,
- steady increase in pump power over several days,
- increased pump flow,
- increased heart rate,
- shortness of breath, or
- redness or oozing at the wound site in the abdomen.

How Do I Take Care of the Driveline?

The driveline connects the LVAD pump inside the person's body to the controller outside his body. The point of exit from the body can be a source of infection. It is important to take care of the wound site to prevent infection. The health care team teaches you how to care for the line and wound site before the person is released. You get opportunities to practice this under supervision before the person is released from the hospital.

What LVAD-Related Complications Should I Watch For?

In addition to the usual postsurgical problems, you need to look out for these complications related to the LVAD:

- Pump thrombus: Clot formation in the pump results in decreased blood flow through the pump. Taking blood thinners as prescribed prevents pump thrombus. If a clot forms in the pump, the person may be short of breath or have an increased pulse. LVAD indicators of clot include increased pulse pressure and a steady increase in pump power over several days. Another concern with clots is that they can break loose and travel to the brain, causing stroke.
- Bleeding: Preventing pump thrombus requires the use of blood thinners, which may cause bleeding. You should call the health care team if the person notices black tarry stools or blood-tinged urine or is coughing up blood. On rare occasions, people have bleeding in the brain that causes a stroke. Regular tests will help identify any minor, non-obvious source of bleeding.
- LVAD infection: Fever, chills, or redness or oozing at the wound site may indicate infection. Call the health care team for guidance if the person has these symptoms.
- Emotional distress: People who receive an LVAD may experience anxiety, depression, or stress related to their heart condition, the LVAD, or care of the LVAD. See chapter 2 on emotions and heart disease for guidance in helping the person with these emotions.

What Medicines Do People with an LVAD Use After Surgery?

Because an LVAD does not replace a weak heart but simply assists it, the additional help of medicines is continued after the person receives an LVAD. However, the dosage may be changed, depending on the individual situation. If the person has not taken warfarin in the past, it will be added. Chewable aspirin, 325 mg once daily, will be a part of the medicine regimen. You should get a detailed, updated medicine list on the person's release from the hospital.

What Activities Can the Person Do After LVAD Surgery?

The LVAD assists with and improves the pumping function of the heart. As a result, the person has an increased energy and activity level and less shortness of breath, leg swelling, and fatigue. The person should notice improved stamina to continue their daily activities.

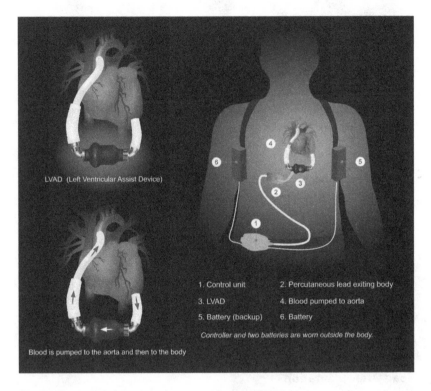

LVAD (Left Ventricular Assist Device)

1. Control unit
3. LVAD
5. Battery (backup)

2. Percutaneous lead exiting body
4. Blood pumped to aorta
6. Battery

Controller and two batteries are worn outside the body.

Blood is pumped to the aorta and then to the body

Figure 5.11. A left ventricular assist device (LVAD) is a pump that assists the pumping function of the heart. It takes blood from the heart and pushes it into the aorta and the rest of the body. © *iStock/Getty Images Plus/Graphic_BKK1979*

However, the person needs to adjust their daily routines. The person and the caregiver have to ensure a power supply to the LVAD at all times. People have to guard the driveline cable so it is not obstructed, even during sleep. You must change dressings at the wound site to prevent infection. Other considerations include:

- Exercise: You should encourage the person to exercise after LVAD surgery. People cannot swim or play contact sports with an LVAD, but they can walk and jog. The physical therapist and cardiac rehabilitation program help identify specific exercises suitable for the person.
- Fluid intake: After years of adjusting to fluid restriction, you and the person have a paradigm shift after LVAD surgery. The LVAD helps the

heart pump more blood, which means that fluid restriction can be eased. You should encourage the person to drink more fluid to avoid dehydration and related dizziness. The doctor may change fluid intake recommendations. You should get instructions on the recommended daily fluid intake and help the person drink adequate fluids. She may be taught to alter the daily intake depending on the LVAD pump flow and pulse index displayed on the controller.

- Travel: People with an LVAD can travel long distances. However, you should discuss travel plans with the health care team and get a letter from them about the LVAD equipment. By showing the letter to security personnel at the airport, the security check will be smooth. You should ensure that there are enough charged batteries to last until the person reaches their destination.
- Driving: The person should not drive for a few weeks after LVAD surgery. Later, the health care team will reassess the condition, and the person may be allowed to drive.
- Sex: People with an LVAD can have sex a few weeks after surgery. Care must be taken to avoid excessive pressure and movement of the driveline at the exit site. Women with an LVAD should not get pregnant.

Heart Transplantation

When a person continues to have cardiomyopathy (weak heart function) despite multiple medicines, surgical procedures, and specialized pacemakers or defibrillators, heart transplantation is considered as a last resort. The person's weak and diseased heart is replaced with a healthy heart from a donor.

Who Is a Candidate for Heart Transplantation?

Heart transplantation is generally offered to people with a weak heart due to:

- coronary artery disease,
- cardiomyopathy of unknown cause,
- heart valve disease, or
- congenital heart defect.

Rarely, it is offered to people with a rare condition called amyloidosis and those with potentially fatal heart rhythm problems for which other treatments have failed.

However, people are not considered for heart transplantation if they:

- are older than seventy;
- have other serious, complex, life-limiting medical conditions (e.g., kidney or liver problems, cancer);
- have an active infection; or
- have an unhealthy lifestyle (e.g., drink alcohol or smoke and are unable to change).

What Are the Risks of Heart Transplantation?

There are risks during and after heart transplantation surgery. Surgical risks include:

- bleeding in the chest,
- infection (especially due to use of certain medicines mentioned later in this chapter),
- blood clots in the legs,
- heart attack,
- stroke, and
- death.

Rejection of the organ is a risk for all people who undergo organ transplantation. The immune system is designed to protect us from foreign objects in the body. Unfortunately, the immune system considers a donated heart a foreign object and tries to attack and destroy it.

To counter this, doctors give medicines to suppress the immune system so that the body accepts the donor heart. Despite the use of these immunosuppressant medicines, one out of ten heart transplant people has a rejection reaction. The doctor treats it aggressively with oral medicines and sometimes with hospital admission and intravenous medicines.

You need to recognize that the person's immune system is always attacking the transplanted heart. This is countered by taking regularly scheduled immunosuppressant medicines. Any lapse in the use of medicines, even a single dose, can give the body's immune system the upper hand and start the process of rejection. This makes it critical that medicine is taken as scheduled, dose after dose, day after day.

You should look for signs of rejection of the transplanted heart, such as:

- fever and flu-like symptoms (e.g., headache, dizziness, general aches, nausea);
- shortness of breath;
- new chest pain or tenderness; or
- tiredness and fatigue.

A heart biopsy is the best way to determine if the body is rejecting the transplanted heart. People are scheduled for a heart biopsy on a regular basis, with the most visits in the first year.

Another problem after heart transplantation is the thickening and hardening of coronary arteries, or cardiac allograft vasculopathy, caused by attacks from the immune system, viral infection, poorly controlled diabetes, cholesterol problems, and smoking. In this condition, the blood supply to the heart muscle decreases, causing heart attack and heart failure, similar to coronary artery disease. The doctor may perform routine tests to assess this condition.

Immunosuppressant medicines used to suppress the body's immune system have side effects (e.g., kidney damage, high cholesterol, diabetes, weak bones, cancers such as non-Hodgkin lymphoma and skin cancer). With the effective suppression of the immune system from these medicines, infection is an ongoing, lifelong concern. You should be attentive to the early signs of infection:

- fever, chills, excessive sweating;
- a wound that does not heal;
- sore throat;
- flu-like symptoms of headaches, fatigue, dizziness;
- frequent urination or burning while urinating;
- pain, tenderness, redness, swelling; or
- symptoms of sinus infection.

How Does the Team Decide Whether Transplantation Is a Good Option?

The health care team meets with the person, family, and caregiver multiple times to understand the disease and its impact on the person. Options such as different medicines, a home health nurse, coronary artery bypass grafting (CABG), valve surgery, and special types of implantable cardioverter defibrillators and left ventricular assist devices are explored. Then the person's other medical conditions, mental health, smoking or alcohol use, family support, and overall well-being are considered. The team reviews the risks of heart transplantation surgery and the care of the person afterward. If the team agrees that heart transplantation will be beneficial, the person is registered (listed) on the transplant list.

What Is My Role After the Person Is on the Transplant List?

People wait for a suitable heart to become available for days to weeks or months, depending on the person's heart condition, blood type, and other factors. You continue to care for the person as before, with medicines, diet, and exercise. Cardiac rehabilitation and a home health nurse may be arranged, if appropriate.

What Happens Once the Person Is on the Transplant List?

When a person dies from a gunshot injury or motor vehicle accident, the family may decide to honor that person by donating his organs. The donor-recipient matching system chooses the best recipient based on several factors (e.g., medical condition, blood type, size of the heart, location of the donor).

The transplantation team notifies the person and caregiver that a heart is available. The person and caregiver need to be reachable to the team twenty-four hours a day, seven days a week. You and the person need to decide immediately whether to take the donor heart or forgo it.

If you decide to take it, the person must reach the hospital within two or three hours. You need to have travel plans and logistics in place. The health care and transplantation teams can help make arrangements and guide you in preparing a travel case with the person's medicines and other items.

What Happens During and After Heart Transplantation?

The preparation for the surgery in the hospital and the care of the person are similar to that of CABG (reviewed earlier in this chapter).

However, postsurgical care for heart transplant people is more intense than that of CABG. The person has very frequent follow-up visits. You should plan to bring the person to the clinic or hospital weekly for the first couple of months. Frequent blood tests, electrocardiograms, and echocardiograms are performed. A heart biopsy, an invasive procedure, is often performed to take a small piece of tissue from the heart and examine it for early signs of rejection.

After the initial period, the doctor visits and testing become less frequent. Once recovered, the person may start to return to routine activities, including exercise, driving, and work. Over time, the person becomes less dependent on you. The person should be encouraged to join a support group for people who have undergone heart transplantation. Cardiac rehabilitation may need to be continued. You should continue to monitor for signs of side effects of medicine, infections, and rejection of the donor heart.

Six

DAY-TO-DAY
CARE ISSUES

I make sure she exercises daily. I think if she continues to exercise, she can overcome heart disease.

—Antonio, whose mother has advanced heart disease

Caregivers can do many things at home to help the person with heart disease keep their heart and body as strong as possible for better quality of life and a longer life. In this chapter, we discuss exercise, diet, fluid and weight management, along with blood pressure and heart rate measurement in patients with heart disease. Additionally, we discuss the physical and emotional safety of a person with heart disease and guide caregivers in navigating these critical issues.

EXERCISE

Over the past few decades, the benefits of exercise have become increasingly apparent. Studies have shown the advantages of regular exercise in all aspects of life, including the prevention of heart disease, treatment of depression, academic success in teens, and community building in seniors.

If the Person Already Has Heart Disease, Is There a Point to Exercising Regularly?

Absolutely! Regular exercise not only helps curb heart problems but also offers many benefits to people at the different stages of heart disease such as:

- a longer life,
- improved quality of life,
- improved blood flow to the heart,
- improved heart function,

- improved use of oxygen,
- faster recovery from surgery,
- fewer hospital visits,
- improved blood pressure,
- improved cholesterol,
- improved blood sugar control in people with diabetes,
- improved symptoms of heart disease over time,
- improved sleep,
- reduced impact of stress, and
- improved maintenance of a healthy weight.

On the other hand, inactive—or sedentary—people with heart disease are worse off, both mentally and physically. They have decreased cognition, high levels of stress, and decreased bone density and muscle mass. Physical inactivity is as deadly as smoking.

Remember that energy begets energy and vice versa. For each day of inactivity, people with heart disease lose 1 percent of their exercise capacity, so it is important to create and stick to an exercise regimen.

Some people may be out of breath or have chest pain and thus may be reluctant to exercise, but it is crucial that they try to exercise as much as their health allows. You should act as a cheerleader to get the person to start and continue a good exercise routine to the extent that their health allows.

You may also play the role of exercise buddy and participate in the exercise routine with the person.

What If the Person Has Not Been Active in the Past?

Exercise benefits everyone with heart disease in at least some of the ways mentioned above, regardless of their previous activity level. In fact, those who are the least active when starting an exercise program seem to benefit the most from it.

People who have never exercised before should do a supervised exercise routine in a formal cardiac rehabilitation program before they can exercise safely at home.

Remember that daily household chores do not count as exercise. One has to set aside a time to perform planned activity that involves repetitive physical movement.

How Does a Person with Heart Disease Start an Exercise Routine?

The ideal way to start an exercise routine is to enroll in a cardiac rehabilitation program.

Doctors refer people to these programs, in which they exercise three times a week for twelve weeks under the supervision of a trained professional. In each session, they exercise for thirty minutes, with a warm-up beforehand and a cooldown afterward. The professional monitors the person's heart rate, blood pressure, and any symptoms with exercise.

At the beginning of the program, a baseline is set for each person, depending on individual situations and needs. The intensity of the exercise is increased or decreased according to the person's comfort. Over time, the person gradually does more intense exercise for longer periods.

At the end of the program, the professional prescribes an exercise type, intensity, and duration that can be safely performed at home. They may also advise people about symptoms to watch for and conditions for which a physician should be consulted.

Supervised exercise programs have proven to be hugely successful and are highly recommended to improve physical and mental health. Unfortunately, these programs remain underused, with only 15 percent of eligible people referred to them. Talk to the doctor about referral and enrollment in cardiac rehabilitation.

We Cannot Enroll in a Cardiac Rehabilitation Program for Logistical Reasons. Can the Person Exercise at Home?

It is advisable to consult the doctor before the person starts unsupervised exercise at home if she:

- had a heart attack recently;
- has not engaged in regular exercise before;
- wants to do more than low-intensity exercise; or
- has chest pain, shortness of breath, or palpitations with minimal exercise.

In these situations, the doctor may perform an exercise test to establish safe limits for exercise.[1]

A typical exercise routine at home should include three phases: warm-up, training, and cooldown.

Warm-Up

The warm-up is five to ten minutes of very low-intensity exercise. In this stage, the person stretches and relaxes her muscles, increases blood flow to the body, and gets ready for the next phase.

Training Phase

The training phase is the main component of the exercise routine. In this phase, the person does an aerobic activity that suits her—such as jogging, walking, swimming, or bicycling—five days a week. Ideally, she gets thirty minutes of aerobic exercise, but depending on her condition, she may break it down into three ten-minute walks or two fifteen-minute walks. An ideal exercise intensity is where the person is able to talk while exercising.

Cooldown

During cooldown, the person continues the aerobic exercise for another five to ten minutes but at a much lower intensity.

Encourage the person to gradually increase the exercise intensity and duration. To get the most benefit, ensure that she exercises for at least 2.5 hours a week.

Strength training should be done twice a week. She should lift one-, two-, or five-pound weights but never exceed ten pounds. If she strains while lifting weights, encourage her to reduce the total weight. It is advisable to teach her the correct technique before she begins weight training.

Ensure adequate hydration during exercise. In case of a break from the exercise routine, she should get back into it gradually.

She Can Exercise for Only Five Minutes at a Time. Should She Continue the Routine?

Absolutely! Every group of people benefits from exercise, regardless of their initial exercise capacity.

The key is to start slow and build up over time. If she can exercise for only five minutes before getting tired, start there, try to get to 5.5 minutes the next week, and build from there week by week. In these situations, consider walking a form of exercise. Some people with arthritis prefer to walk in the pool since it is easier on the joints.

Walking is easy on the body and doesn't require special equipment. The person should wear comfortable clothing and stay hydrated. You should walk with the person for motivation and companionship.

The person should rest or stop exercising if any of the following occur:

- chest pain,
- breathlessness,
- irregular heartbeat,
- lightheadedness,
- dizziness, or
- palpitations.

The person may get tired more easily and take longer to perform than you expect. You should recognize and account for this when scheduling activities.

Is There an Ideal Time of Day to Exercise?

The person should exercise at the time of day she feels most energetic. After a good night's rest, most people feel most energetic in the morning.

The person should avoid exercising in the first hour after a meal because the blood flow is directed to the stomach, making it difficult to exercise. Encourage her to exercise indoors when it is warmer than 80 degrees Fahrenheit (27 degrees Celsius) or cooler than 40 degrees Fahrenheit (four degrees Celsius), as well as after a snowstorm or if there is heavy smog.

What Is the Ideal Intensity of Exercise?

As mentioned previously, the person should be able to talk while exercising. If she cannot, advise her to slow down. If she feels tired during exercise, she should rest and restart at a lower intensity when she is ready. Build up the exercise intensity and duration gradually.

Also, the person will have good days and bad days. On a good day, the person is able to perform more exercise and activities of daily living. You should encourage this and recognize that, on other days, the person may have low energy and be unable to exercise as much. Over time, you will better understand this ebb and flow, which is normal in heart disease.

Should I Monitor the Person's Heart Rate When She Exercises at Home? What Is the Target Heart Rate?

In general, the ideal heart rate is a range, just like ideal height and weight. No one number is the ideal heart rate for all people. Most importantly, their disease as well as their medicines affect the heart rate. So exercise routines based on heart rate may not be suitable for people with advanced heart disease.

Most people benefit from having a tailored exercise regimen developed by a professional after they complete a cardiac rehabilitation program. In these programs, a trained professional assesses their exercise against symptoms and changes in blood pressure and heart rate. People benefit from an exercise routine based on these multiple variables rather than on the single parameter of target heart rate. In the absence of cardiac rehabilitation, the person should be able to talk while exercising. If she cannot, it is advisable to slow down. If she feels tired during exercise or experiences any of the symptoms mentioned above, she should rest, restart at a lower intensity, and then build up the exercise intensity and duration gradually.

If the Person Is on the Transplant List, Should She Exercise?

Yes, the person should continue to exercise even if she is on the list for a heart transplant.

People who continue to be active before a heart transplant recover faster after it. Even in an intensive care unit, depending on the person's symptoms, some activity is recommended.

Even if the person has a ventricular assist device, exercise under supervision is possible and recommended. A trained professional can guide her to continue to exercise safely around its wires, battery packs, and other components.

After a heart transplant, exercises should first be performed under supervision, and people can continue to exercise unsupervised at home once they feel comfortable.

What Symptoms Should I Watch for During Exercise?

If the person develops chest pain, shortness of breath, lightheadedness, or an irregular heartbeat, she should stop exercising and see if the symptoms go away. If they do, write down the exercise she was doing, how long she had been doing it, the time of day, what she experienced, and how long it took for the symptoms to pass. Share these details with the doctor.

If symptoms do not go away, contact your doctor immediately or call 911. People who previously had chest pain should always carry nitroglycerin pills with them. Changes in chest pain intensity or duration may point to worsening of the heart disease.

Can a Person with Advanced Heart Disease Do Other Forms of Exercise? How About Yoga?

Yes! Yoga and weight or resistance training are great options.

Weight and Resistance Training

Weight and resistance training are recommended for people with heart disease. The person's cardiologist/physical therapist may be able to offer guidance regarding any specific restrictions. In general, weight and resistance training should be done twice a week. The person may increase the number of repetitions but not the weight. The maximum weight that a person with advanced heart disease should lift is ten pounds. She should not bear down or strain during weight lifting. It is important that she learn proper form from a professional trainer.

Yoga

Hot yoga is not advisable due to the high likelihood of a large drop in blood pressure, which can be dangerous for a person with advanced heart disease. Other forms of yoga may be undertaken, although currently there is little scientific evidence to support or restrict its practice.

How Can I Know if the Person Is Overexerting Herself?

If you notice that the person is experiencing these symptoms during exercise, advise her to slow down or stop and seek medical advice:

- shortness of breath that prevents the person from completing a sentence;
- ongoing shortness of breath that does not improve when she stops exercising;
- dizziness or lightheadedness during exercise;
- chest pain or tightness;
- pain in the arms, shoulders, neck, or jaw;
- palpitations; or
- unusual or extreme fatigue.

How Can I Motivate a Person to Exercise?

Exercising with a companion is always enjoyable. You should join the person during the exercise routine. This will help you ensure safety, monitor progress, and offer support. People who know that they have a partner in their journey tend to stick to and progress in their exercise program.

Many tools and apps are available to motivate people to exercise. One example is Map My Fitness, a free app that records the person's exercise over time. The results can be shared with you. Another app for iPhone users is Cardiio. Pedometers and exercise apps like Strava can help track the person's aerobic capacity.

Should Any Person with Advanced Heart Disease Not Exercise?

Most people with heart disease benefit from exercise, with a few exceptions:

- People with narrowed aortic valves are at risk with exercise.
- People with hypertrophic cardiomyopathy (thickening of the heart muscle) may experience side effects when exercising.
- If a person has had severe heart rhythm problems while exercising, it may happen again.

These people should not exercise before having a detailed discussion with their doctor.

Furthermore, if the person experiences chest pain, shortness of breath, dizziness, or loss of consciousness with exercise, she must talk to her doctor before continuing.

How Can I as a Caregiver Fit Exercise into My Routine?

It is important for you to continue to care for your own health while taking care of the person. There is always the opportunity to go for a light jog with the person on a regular basis.

Other Creative Ways of Including More Activity in Your Day

- Use the stairs instead of the elevator.
- Park far away from destinations and walk the rest of the way, if weather permits.
- If you work, incorporate exercise into your lunch hour.
- Run or hit the gym when the person is resting or sleeping.

There are many ways to work exercise into your daily life, no matter your situation.

DIET

In people with advanced heart disease, the heart muscle is damaged and cannot pump blood effectively. Although this is a chronic condition with no cure, the symptoms can be managed.

Increased body weight and fluid retention can lead to negative outcomes in these people, so it is essential to:

- maintain a healthy weight,
- eat a balanced diet,
- limit salt intake, and
- restrict fluid intake.

Are Weight Considerations for People with Advanced Heart Disease Different from Those of the Rest of Us Who Are Trying to Prevent Heart Disease?

Yes. In addition to the usual concerns about obesity, weight has an additional dimension for people with advanced heart disease.

Fluid-Related Weight Gain

In people with heart failure, any sudden increase in weight is a concern because it may indicate fluid retention. Fluid-related weight (also called water weight) gain can lead to hospitalization.

Non-Fluid-Related Weight Gain

This is also cause for concern because it can lead to high blood pressure, stroke, and other cardiac events.

You should focus on water weight in the short term and overall weight for the long-term health of the person.

What Is the Ideal Weight for People with Advanced Heart Disease?

It is critical for the person to maintain a healthy body weight. Losing weight can be difficult for people with advanced heart disease. However, with a disciplined exercise and diet routine, they may be able to achieve their ideal body weight over time.

You play the role of coach and cheerleader in helping the person maintain these lifestyle changes.

People with advanced heart disease should maintain a baseline weight at which they are most comfortable without feeling tired or short of breath or having chest pain. Any sudden increase in weight over two or three days may indicate water weight. If the person has been hospitalized for heart failure, weight at hospital release is a good indication of the target body weight.

How Should a Person with Advanced Heart Disease Maintain the Ideal Body Weight?

Because many people with advanced heart disease have limited exercise capacity, maintaining their ideal body weight can be challenging.

The following guidelines can prevent weight gain:

- The number of calories consumed should match the number of calories burned each day. You should encourage the use of a smart phone app like LoseIt! or MyFitnessPal to track the person's caloric intake.
- People should give food their undivided attention. When people are distracted (e.g., watching television), they tend to eat more. You should eat with the person and minimize distractions at the dinner table.
- Set aside forty-five minutes for dinner so the person can eat slowly. People should put down their knife and fork after each bite and count how many times they chew before swallowing. Because the brain begins to register feelings of fullness only after twenty minutes, eating quickly can easily lead to overeating. You can model this behavior for the person.
- Discourage the person from overeating. According to a wise Chinese saying, "Your stomach should be one-third solid, one-third liquid, and one-third air."
- Use small plates. Having less on a plate helps with portion control.
- Keep pots and serving platters away from the dinner table so the person has to get up for a second serving.
- Be mindful of the liquid calories the person consumes in soft drinks, alcohol, and juices.
- Watch the person's sugar intake.
- Eliminate all junk food from the house; if it is not there, the person cannot eat it. You should place an embargo on junk food.
- Eat out less often. When eating out, follow the guidelines below.

What Precautions Should We Take While Eating Out?

People are at risk for consuming more calories and sodium than usual when they eat out. Following these simple guidelines will help reduce their overall calorie and sodium intake:

- Go to restaurants the person is familiar with; avoid national chain and fast food restaurants.
- Choose the restaurant ahead of time. The person and you can review the menu online to ensure that the restaurant offers options that meet dietary requirements.
- Select dishes with vegetables as the main ingredient.
- Ask the server what ingredients the dish contains and how it's prepared (e.g., fried or grilled).
- Ask for alterations and substitutions, such as less salt. Most chefs are happy to accommodate such requests.
- When ordering a salad, ask for the dressing on the side to control how much the person consumes.
- Do not touch the bread basket.
- If the person orders a drink, ask for the smallest size.
- The person should not feel obligated to drink a full glass of water every time the server refills it.
- People who drink alcohol should limit themselves to two drinks per day.
- Be mindful of sugar content in nonalcoholic beverages such as tea and soda.
- If the restaurant's serving is large, bring a takeout container or ask for one before you start eating. Divide the food between the person's plate and the container, and take the rest home. Alternatively, you can split the dish with the person to limit portion size and caloric intake.
- If the person wants dessert, suggest a fruit dish.

How Do I Limit Sodium Intake?

Sodium is an essential element found in most food sources and a major component of table salt/common salt. For people with heart failure, sodium management is critical. The more sodium they consume, the more water their body retains. This increases the chance of weight gain, breathing difficulties, and hospitalization. Sodium intake affects blood pressure.

All this makes it critical to limit sodium intake to less than 2,300 mg per day. Here are some tips to help manage salt intake:

- Of the salt that we consume from food, 70 percent comes from food prepared outside the home, such as canned and processed foods, takeout, and restaurant meals. Freshly prepared homemade meals are ideal. You can take on the role of chef or assistant chef to encourage home cooking.
- Watch for these high-sodium foods and avoid making them part of the meal: bread and rolls, cold cuts and cured meats, pizza, canned soups and vegetables, pickles, snacks, and sandwiches.
- Avoid condiments such as ketchup, mayonnaise, and soy sauce. If the person must use condiments, choose reduced-salt versions such as reduced-sodium soy sauce and ketchup.
- When eating out, view the menu online in advance and choose from the lower-salt options. Discuss low-salt substitutes with the server or chef. Remember that Chinese food contains excessive salt.
- Remember that sea salt contains the same amount of sodium as regular salt. Buy low-sodium salt options available at the supermarket.
- Read food labels and understand how much sodium and calories foods contain (see instructions below).

How to Read and Understand Food Labels

Nutrition Facts
Serving Size 3 oz. (85g)
Serving Per Container 2

Amount Per Serving

Calories 200	Calories from Fat 120

	% Daily Value*
Total Fat 15g	**20 %**
Saturated Fat 5g	**28 %**
Trans Fat 3g	
Cholesterol 30mg	**10 %**
Sodium 650mg	**28 %**
Total Carbohydrate 30g	**10 %**
Dietary Fiber 0g	**0 %**
Sugars 5g	
Protein 5g	

Vitamin A 5%	•	Vitamin C 2%
Calcium 15%	•	Iron 5%

*Percent Daily Values are based on a 2,000 calorie diet. Your Daily Values may be higher or lower depending on your calorie needs.

	Calories	2,000	2,500
Total Fat	Less than	65g	80g
Sat Fat	Less than	20g	25g
Cholesterol	Less than	300mg	300mg
Sodium	Less than	2,400mg	2,400mg
Total Carbohydrate		300mg	375mg
Dietary Fiber		25g	30g

Figure 6.1. Sample nutrition facts food label for a box of macaroni and cheese. In order to follow sodium and calorie recommendations, it is important to read food labels. © DigitalVision Vectors/Getty Images Plus/mustafahacalaki

In order to follow sodium and calorie recommendations, it is important to read food labels. When reading any food label, start at the top with the serving size. In the example in figure 6.1, one serving is about one-third of a cup. If the person consumes the whole box, he will consume two servings, which will provide 200 calories × 2 = 400 calories and 650 mg × 2 = 1,300 mg of sodium.

It is critical to do these calculations for all the food and drinks the person consumes. Caregivers can play a big role in encouraging people to get into this habit.

How Can I Help Manage Fluid Intake?

Fluid management is critical in advanced heart disease. Typically, people are advised to restrict their fluids to 1.5 to 2 liters per day. However, there are some key considerations:

- If the person is thirsty, encourage drinking water. Thirst indicates dehydration.
- If the person complains of lightheadedness and the blood pressure is unusually low, the person might be dehydrated. Encourage drinking more water.
- Count coffee, tea, soda, juices, wine, beer, and other drinks toward the daily fluid limit.
- If the person drinks from a bottle or glass, he does not have to finish it if he is not thirsty.

What Is the Best Diet for People with Heart Disease? The Mediterranean Diet? Keto Diet? South Beach Diet?

People and family members get confused due to conflicting recommendations from different specialists. Instead of following a specific diet, consider these evidence-based, healthy, and balanced food principles:

- Eat more vegetables, especially red, yellow, and orange ones such as carrots, sweet potatoes, red peppers, and acorn squash. They are high in nutritional value and low in calories.
- Use spinach instead of lettuce in your salads.
- Eat more broccoli and asparagus.
- Eat more fruit; strawberries, raspberries, blueberries, and cranberries are good options.
- Eat more nuts; almonds and walnuts are good options.

- Eat more whole grains; whole wheat, quinoa, barley, and farro are good options.
- Avoid foods made with refined, white flour like white bread, muffins, frozen waffles, cornbread, doughnuts, biscuits, quick breads, cakes, pies, egg noodles, buttered popcorn, crackers, and high-fat snacks.
- Have oatmeal for breakfast.
- Have fish twice a week; salmon, herring, and mackerel are good choices.
- Avoid trans fats (may be labeled as "hydrogenated vegetable oil" on packaging).
- Use extra virgin olive oil, canola oil, vegetable oil, and nut oils. Flavor your salads with olive oil and vinegar/lemon instead of packaged dressings.
- Avoid whole milk, creamers, butter, margarine, lard, bacon fat, gravy, and cream sauces.
- Avoid red meat. If the person wants to eat meat, choose lean meats and cuts (e.g., poultry without the skin).
- Although vegetables and fruits are highly recommended, avoid foods such as coconut products, vegetables with creamy sauces, fried or breaded vegetables, canned fruit in heavy syrup, and frozen fruit with added sugar.

What Are the Best Sources of Protein and Carbs?

Adequate protein intake is a concern for people with advanced heart disease, especially when they are trying to avoid meat and eggs. The following alternative sources of protein are recommended:

- plant-based proteins such as flax seed, walnuts, and soybeans;
- soy or tofu burgers;
- legumes such as beans, peas, and lentils (give preference to dark-colored beans such as black or kidney beans);
- fish like salmon, mackerel, and herring (good sources of protein and heart-healthy omega-3 fatty acids);
- canola oil for cooking;
- low-fat dairy products; and
- lean meat or poultry (least recommended).

While the person avoids carbohydrates from refined sugar and refined white flour, the following alternative sources of carbohydrate are recommended: brown rice, oatmeal, sweet potatoes, quinoa, barley, and farro.

Is Alcohol Safe for People with Heart Disease?

Caregivers tend to rightly be concerned about alcohol intake. Heavy alcohol use has a catastrophic effect on the heart; it causes a weakness of the heart called "alcoholic cardiomyopathy."[2]

The type of alcohol consumed (beer, wine, or liquor) does not alter this negative outcome. In people with heavy alcohol use, caregivers need help from Alcoholics Anonymous and other support groups to help the person quit alcohol.

One study showed that moderate alcohol consumption—no more than two drinks per day—decreases the risk of heart failure and lengthens the life span in advanced heart disease.[3] However, other studies have not shown the same benefit.

The only evidence-based advice one can offer is that abstainers should not start drinking and drinkers should limit their intake to two drinks per day. You can help track the person's alcohol intake.

Is Caffeine Safe for People with Heart Disease?

Based on several well-conducted studies, drinking a moderate amount of coffee does not seem to affect people with heart disease negatively.[4]

How Can the Person Eat More Fruits and Vegetables?

Everyone, including people with heart disease, should eat five servings of fruits and vegetables each day. The following well-established tricks help people eat more fruits and vegetables:

- Wash and cut fresh vegetables and place them in a visible location in the fridge.
- Use carrots and celery as snacks.
- Wash fruits and keep in a bowl in a prominent place in the kitchen.
- Eat entrees that have vegetables as the main ingredient.
- Cook with tomato sauces rather than cream-based ones.
- When shopping for groceries, buy enough vegetables and fruit for the week.

Where Can I Find Heart-Healthy Recipes?

Here are some good websites for appropriate recipes:

- recipes.heart.org
- recipes.heart.org/en/collections/lifestyles/vegetarian
- cookinglight.com/eating-smart/nutrition-101/heart-healthy-vegetarian -recipes
- foodnetwork.com/healthy/photos/favorite-heart-healthy-recipes

DRY WEIGHT AND FLUID WEIGHT

It is important for people with advanced heart disease to weigh themselves at the same time of the day every day. Place a bathroom scale with large display numbers on a hard, flat surface. Most people find it convenient to weigh themselves in the morning after using the bathroom and before eating or getting dressed.

The person should use the same scale daily and weigh themselves either with no clothes or the same number of clothes. It is difficult to remember weight, so it is critical to write it down. Use the chart below to keep a log of weight measurements.

The weight at which the person's body has no extra fluid is called the "dry" weight. Thus, people may have minor fluctuations from the dry weight. Weight may vary if a different scale is used (e.g., at the doctor's office). The person may be given a daily limit on fluid intake. If so, it is important to track daily fluid intake and ensure that the person does not exceed this limit.

Date	Weight	Blood pressure	Heart rate	Short of breath?	Foot or leg swelling or abdomen bloating?	How do you feel? Other symptoms?
				Yes/No	Yes/No	
				Yes/No	Yes/No	
				Yes/No	Yes/No	
				Yes/No	Yes/No	
				Yes/No	Yes/No	
				Yes/No	Yes/No	

Tip for Tracking Fluid Intake

Some people and caregivers track fluid intake by filling a bottle with the amount of water equal to the daily fluid limit (e.g., 48 ounces), and then drink water from it. Every time the person drinks fluid in any form, the same amount of water is emptied from the bottle. When the bottle is empty, the daily fluid limit is reached. Remember that soups, ice cream, yogurt, pudding, and gelatin (Jell-O) are considered fluids.

When Should You Call the Doctor's Office or 911?

If the person gains more than two pounds in a day or more than five pounds in a week, call the doctor's office. It may be an early sign that the person is retaining fluid, so early treatment may help him avoid a hospital stay. The health care team may also ask the person and caregiver to use water pills (diuretics) based on weight changes.

If the person gains more than two pounds in a day and is extremely short of breath even at rest, call 911.

When you contact the doctor's office, be prepared to answer the following questions:

- What is the person's name?
- What is the person's date of birth?
- Who is the person's primary cardiologist?
- Who is the nurse you generally talk with about these matters?
- What is the person's usual weight?
- What is the person's blood pressure and heart rate?
- Does the person have chest pain, shortness of breath, or other symptoms?
- What medicines does the person take regularly? Does he take any medicines on an as-needed basis? Has he taken them recently? Any recent changes in medicines? Has he used any natural supplements or over-the-counter medicines recently?
- Has the person been hospitalized for similar problems in the past?
- Has the person missed or run out of prescribed medicines?
- Has the person been adhering to fluid restrictions?
- Any recent increase in salt or alcohol intake?
- Any recent outing to a restaurant?

What Tests and Treatments Will the Doctor Likely Recommend?

You may be asked to bring the person to the doctor's office for an in-person examination. If the person has a pacemaker, defibrillator, or monitor, the doctor will check it. She may recommend hospitalization or evaluate the problem in the clinic. The following tests may be conducted:

- blood pressure check to see if there is an increase or decrease in blood pressure;
- blood tests to identify any anemia or electrolyte imbalances and assess kidney and thyroid function;
- chest radiograph to look for fluid in the lungs;
- electrocardiogram to check heart rhythm and rate; or
- echocardiogram, an ultrasound test discussed in chapter 5, to check heart pumping and identify any previous heart attacks or valve problems.

At-home treatment recommendations may include:

- fluid and salt restriction,
- increase in water pills,
- better blood pressure control, and
- change in other medicines.

BLOOD PRESSURE

In addition to daily weight, people with advanced heart disease must track their daily blood pressure. Many good automated, upper-arm-cuff blood pressure machines are sold for home use. They can be found at any pharmacy, where a pharmacist can help choose the machine with the right-sized cuff.

After buying the blood pressure machine, take it to the next doctor's appointment. The doctor or nurse can ensure that you are using it correctly and that the machine gives accurate results.

Blood pressure should be measured at the same time every day. Most people find it convenient to check it in the morning about an hour after taking their medicines. The person should sit still for five minutes with the back straight, legs uncrossed, feet on the floor, and arm supported on the table before measuring it. The cuff should be applied directly over the skin and not over clothes.

Blood pressure is recorded as two measurements: systolic and diastolic. Systolic blood pressure is the top number, and diastolic blood pressure is the bottom number. They are conveyed as millimeters of mercury (mm Hg). The recommended blood pressure is less than 140/80 mm Hg, but the doctor will identify the target blood pressure for the person. However, do not replace these numbers by your assessment as "normal," "high," or "low." Record blood pressure on the chart provided previously as 124/82, 116/78, and so on.

If one blood pressure reading is very different from the usual one, wait five minutes and retake it. A difference of as much as 10 mm Hg between the right and left arm is normal.

When Should I Call the Doctor's Office or 911?

It is important to track blood pressure after any changes have been made in medicines. If a large change in blood pressure occurs, call the doctor's office. If the blood pressure is above 180/120 mm Hg repeatedly, call the doctor's office immediately.

If the person has chest pain, shortness of breath, changes in vision, slurred speech, or headaches along with blood pressure above 180/120 mm Hg, call 911. If it is below 90/60 mm Hg and that is unusual for the person and he is feeling lightheaded and dizzy, call the doctor's office. If he is fainting or nearly fainting, call 911.

When you contact the doctor's office, be prepared to answer the following questions:

- What is the person's name?
- What is the person's date of birth?
- Who is the person's primary cardiologist?
- Who is the nurse you generally talk with about these matters?
- What is the person's heart rate?
- What is the person's usual blood pressure at home?
- Does the person have fluctuations in blood pressure?
- Does the person have chest pain, shortness of breath, blurry vision, light-headedness, dizziness, or other symptoms?
- What medicines does the person take regularly? Does he take any medicines on an as-needed basis? Has he taken them recently? Any recent changes in medicines? Has he used any natural supplements or over-the-counter medicines recently?
- Has the person been hospitalized for similar problems in the past?
- Has the person reliably taken the prescribed medicines?
- Has the person had any other illnesses recently?

What Tests and Treatment Plans Will the Doctor Likely Recommend?

You may be asked to bring the person to the doctor's office for an in-person examination. If the person has chest pain or pressure, shortness of breath, or vision changes, hospitalization may be recommended. Alternatively, evaluation and treatment in the clinic may suffice. The following tests may be conducted:

- blood pressure check to see if the change can be verified,
- blood tests to look for conditions such as anemia and check kidney function,
- electrocardiogram to check heart rhythm and effect of blood pressure on the heart,
- urine test to look for blood in the urine, and
- ultrasound to check the kidneys.

Treatment recommendations may include:

- fluid and salt restriction,
- change in medicines to improve blood pressure, and
- follow-up visit to check blood pressure and heart rate and conduct an electrocardiogram.

HEART RATE

In addition to daily weight and blood pressure, people must track their heart rate (same as pulse rate). Blood pressure machines also measure heart rate. Some people use a pulse oximeter or smart watch to measure their heart rate.

Normal heart rate for adults is 60 to 100 beats per minute. It is important to know the person's usual resting heart rate. Heart rate and blood pressure should be measured at the same time.

When Should I Call the Doctor's Office or 911?

If the heart rate is repeatedly 30 beats per minute above the person's usual rate, call the doctor's office.

If the heart rate is below 50 beats a minute and the person is lightheaded, dizzy, short of breath, or fainting, call 911.

When you call the doctor's office, be prepared to answer the following questions:

- What is the person's name?
- What is the person's date of birth?

- Who is the person's primary cardiologist?
- Who is the nurse you generally talk with about these matters?
- What is the person's usual heart rate at home?
- What is the person's blood pressure?
- Does the person have lightheadedness, dizziness, fainting, chest pain, shortness of breath, or palpitations?
- What medicines does the person take regularly? Does he take any medicines on an as-needed basis? Has he taken them recently? Any recent changes in medicines? Has he used any natural supplements or over-the-counter medicines recently?
- Has the person reliably taken the prescribed medicines?
- Does the person have atrial fibrillation? Any other heart rhythm abnormality?
- Does the person have a pacemaker or defibrillator?
- Has the person had any other illness recently?

What Tests and Treatment Plans Will the Doctor Likely Recommend?

You may be asked to bring the person to the doctor's office for an in-person examination. If the person has a pacemaker or a defibrillator, the doctor will check it. If the person is lightheaded, dizzy, or fainting, hospitalization may be recommended.

If the person has an abnormal heart rhythm, hospitalization may be recommended so he can receive intravenous medicine or electrical cardioversion. Alternatively, evaluation and treatment in the clinic may suffice. The following tests may be conducted:

- blood pressure check to see if it changes with the change in heart rate;
- blood tests to identify conditions such as anemia and check kidney function;
- electrocardiogram to check heart rhythm and rate; or
- one-, two-, fourteen-, or twenty-eight-day heart monitor to check for variations in heart rate.

Treatment recommendations may include:

- change in medicines to improve heart rate control or
- pacemaker for very low heart rate.

PHYSICAL SAFETY

Advanced heart disease poses unique challenges to the physical safety of patients.

Falls

Falls at home are common in older people, with nearly a third of seniors experiencing fall-related injury each year. In heart patients, low blood pressure or slow or fast heart rhythms can make patients dizzy and pass out. Furthermore, many heart patients are in an older age group and frail. Patients and caregivers need to take precautions, such as:

- Recognize that a person with balance issues or muscle weakness may be at increased risk for falls. Talk to your doctor about a formal fall risk assessment.
- The doctor can review the person's medicine list for any medicines that can cause dizziness, muscle weakness, drowsiness, or imbalance and make changes.
- Go through the house and identify tripping hazards (e.g., clutter, books, shoes, small pieces of furniture, cords, rugs, frayed carpeting). These hazards need to be cleared or dealt with appropriately (e.g., tape rugs to the floor).
- Rearrange furniture to provide adequate walking space.
- Ensure that all areas of the house are well lit. Nightlights should be placed within reach and function properly. Many falls occur when one gets up in the middle of the night to use the bathroom.
- If the person depends on furniture or walls for support, he can consider using a cane or walker.
- Use rails when going up and down the stairs.
- Consider installing a chairlift to help the person go up and down the stairs.
- Wear nonslip socks; slippers with rubber or no-slip bottoms; flat, thin-soled shoes; and other such footwear on smooth surfaces.
- Install stability bars in showers and near toilets the person uses. Nonslip rubber mats in the shower decrease the chance of falls in the bathtub.
- If the person has difficulty getting in and out of the bathtub or on and off the toilet, talk to your doctor about prescribing a special tub chair, bench, or raised toilet seat.

- The person may faint while getting out of a hot tub or after coming out from a prolonged hot shower. To prevent this, ensure that the water temperature is set for no more than 104 degrees Fahrenheit and the shower lasts no more than fifteen minutes to avoid low blood pressure and related fainting.
- Regular exercise improves muscle and bone strength, which also decreases the risk of falls. Walking, water exercise, and tai chi improve strength, balance, and coordination and prevent falls. A physical therapist can help structure a specific exercise program to encourage the person to exercise regularly and safely.
- Enroll the person in one of the special classes offered at many centers on ways to prevent falls.
- Use a bracelet or necklace medical alert with which the person can alert medical services in the event of a fall to eliminate the need to look for a phone.
- Some medical alert systems automatically detect falls and notify emergency services. People who have fallen before may benefit from such an "auto-alert" system.
- Replace a landline with a cellphone or a cordless phone so that the person does not have to rush to the phone, a common cause of falls in older people.
- If the person has sudden urges to urinate, a health care provider may be able to reduce these symptoms. Such patients are at increased risk for falls when they try to rush to the bathroom to prevent an accident.
- Make an appointment for an annual eye exam to ensure good vision and help prevent falls due to an inability to see clearly. Replace eyeglasses as needed.
- The trade organization National Association of Home Builders offers certified aging-in-place specialists who can design and modify homes to make them safer for older adults. Call 800-368-5242 or visit nahb.org to locate an expert in your area.

Fires

People with advanced heart disease may need to use supplemental oxygen at home, which poses a fire hazard. Ensure the presence of working smoke detectors in the house, and schedule battery changes twice a year. Avoid open flames near the oxygen tank. No smokers should be allowed near the person using supplemental oxygen, especially not with a lit cigarette.

Check electrical appliances for frayed cords and reduce fire hazards due to malfunctioning or improperly grounded appliances. Never leave candles burning in an empty room. Ensure that heaters are at least three feet away from anything inflammable (e.g., curtains, bedding, furniture).

Poisoning

Older people with advanced heart disease take multiple medicines. Due to age, memory loss, confusion, and complex medical regimens, accidental drug overdoses are a distinct possibility. Caregivers can help prevent this by helping the person fill their pillbox each week, training and monitoring for appropriate use of medicines, and insisting on larger, easier-to-read labels. Medicines should be taken in well-lit areas, and bring all pill bottles to doctor visits so the doctor knows the medicines the person is taking. Inappropriate medicine use is a common cause of patient suffering and even death. Appropriate medicine use is further described in chapter 7.

Crime

Crimes against older people, both online and offline, have increased recently. Caregivers should educate and protect older people against it. Ways to prevent this can be found in other authoritative sources and are beyond the scope of this book. The following emergency numbers should be kept in a well-lit place for quick reference:

- 911,
- Poison Control: 800-222-1222,
- caregiver's phone number,
- family member or friend to call in case of emergency, and
- health care provider's office number.

Preventing Infections

Older people have weak immune systems, making them highly susceptible to infection. People with heart disease may be further compromised in their ability to fight infection, especially if they have other medical issues.

This makes it critical to prevent infections by following some basic infection-control practices. The caregiver is generally in charge of implementing these practices.

Urinary tract infections, influenza, pneumonia, and skin infections are the most common infections and can spread into the bloodstream and cause sepsis.

Controlling Infections at Home

Hand washing is the best way to prevent spread of infection. This is especially important while preparing food and before physical contact with the patient and their medical equipment. The caregiver should use proper hand-washing techniques after using the bathroom, lathering for at least twenty seconds. If the hands are not visibly dirty, using alcohol-based sanitizers is adequate.

One should feel comfortable asking all visitors to wash their hands before touching them. This includes visiting nurses, home health aides, physical therapists, and occupational therapists providing care at home.

Loved ones who are sick should avoid visiting people with advanced heart disease. If they do visit, ask them to wear a face mask and gloves to prevent spreading the infection.

Equipment (e.g., urinary catheters, thermometers) should be kept sterilized.

Do not share personal items or toiletries with the person.

If the person has cuts and scratches, clean, cover, and monitor them for signs such as redness, swelling, pain, and oozing.

Caregivers should inspect the person's feet regularly for infection, especially if the person has diabetes, and keep them clean and dry. The caregiver should take over the responsibility of trimming nails if the person is unsteady or frail.

Vaccinate yourself and the person against influenza each fall. The person should receive the pneumonia vaccine every five years. The Centers for Disease Control and Prevention recommend two doses of the shingles vaccine two to six months apart.

Caregivers should be especially careful when caring for open wounds, sores, ports, intravenous lines, and other access sites into the body to prevent infection. Learn to care for these sites from professionals before taking over the responsibility.

A good diet gives the person the necessary nutrients to boost the immune system and fight infection. Caregivers should consider adding berries, green leafy vegetables, and healthy fats to the person's diet.

Stress and anxiety weaken the immune system. Hence, better management of stress decreases the body's susceptibility to infections. See chapter 2 and "Managing Emotions" section in this chapter for ways to manage stress and anxiety.

Regular exercise and physical activity boost the immune system. Encourage the person to be physically active to ward off infections.

Recognizing Signs of Infection

Early detection of infection can lead to prompt treatment and complete recovery. Caregivers play an important role in recognizing subtle signs of infection. Fever greater than 101.5 degrees Fahrenheit, chills or tremors, rapid breathing, palpitations, and dizziness may be early signs of infection. Older people with advanced heart disease may show atypical signs of infection such as decreased appetite, change in alertness level and mental status, confusion, hallucinations, agitation, or an extraordinary change in energy levels. In cases of pneumonia, cough with or without sputum, chest pain, and increased difficulty breathing may be noted. With urinary tract infection, burning during urination, change in frequency or volume of urination, or incontinence may be the initial complaint. Wound infection is suspected if there is increased redness, swelling, or oozing of fluid from the wound site or itching or pain at the site. Abdominal pain, nausea, vomiting, and diarrhea may indicate infection of the gastrointestinal tract with virus or bacteria. Call the doctor's office if the person has any of the following signs:

- a cough that lasts longer than a week;
- a fever lasting longer than forty-eight hours;
- a new rash or swelling in any part of the body;
- discharge from a wound site;
- unexplained agitation, confusion, or hallucinations;
- burning or discomfort during urination;
- a severe headache with fever; or
- trouble breathing.

MANAGING EMOTIONS

Caregivers play a major role in helping people manage the feelings of loss, lack of control, and fear that come with advanced heart disease.

What Feelings and Emotions Do People with Heart Disease Experience?

People with heart disease, especially advanced heart disease, may have negative emotions such as:

- depression,
- anxiety,
- anger,
- loss of control,
- grief,
- loneliness,
- uncertainty, or
- feeling like a burden to others.

These feelings are common in people with heart disease, with up to 70 percent feeling depressed at some point during the course of their disease. However, in addition to their psychological toll, these emotions affect people in many other ways.

Depression and anxiety can lead to an imbalance of hormones, which can in turn worsen blood pressure and heart failure. People with negative emotions may have low energy, poor appetite, and a disrupted sleep pattern. Moreover, depressed people may not take their medicines on time and fail to seek medical help when needed. As a result, they may be hospitalized often and have poor survival rates.

On the other hand, people with a positive outlook are better able to manage their disease, stick to diet and exercise recommendations, and adhere to their medical regimen.

What Is My Role in Recognizing Negative Emotions?

People with heart disease tend to minimize these symptoms or attribute them to other factors such as heart failure, advancing age, or normal aging processes. You have a critical role in recognizing these emotions and helping the person manage them appropriately.

How Can I Recognize These Emotions?

As someone in daily contact with the person, you can recognize if these feelings and moods have lasted longer than two weeks.

You may notice the person feeling down, withdrawing from others, and losing interest in activities they once cherished. Some may complain of fatigue and spend more time in bed. Others may show an unusual loss of interest in food or sex. In the worse cases, the person may talk about hopelessness or even consider suicide. All these signs indicate the possibility of depression.

How Can I Identify Anxiety in the Person?

If the person appears tense and restless, worries excessively, and seems fearful for longer than two weeks, they may have anxiety.

Can I Do Anything Besides Contacting the Doctor?

Yes. In addition to recognizing the signs of depression, anxiety, anger, and fear, you can help the person cope with their condition, symptoms, and behavior.

Talking about feelings is very powerful. Talking out loud about concerns makes them feel less overwhelming and more manageable.

- Ask the person to identify their feelings about their symptoms and heart condition. Use statements like, "I have heard that people with heart disease go through phases of anxiety, depression, and hopelessness about their life. Have you had such thoughts?" Alternatively, you can use more open-ended questions such as "You seem on edge these days. Do you want to talk about it?" This invitation will open the dialogue.
- Give the person space to explore. Listen. This may give him time to reflect on his feelings.
- Refrain from judgment or trying to change how the person feels. Having a trusted friend to listen to how he feels can help him reduce stress and feel greater ease. Validate and normalize his feelings.
- If you help the person identify how he feels, he can quickly change his behavior when he is in a rut and can ask for help without shame or fear. He can get the support he needs and improve his sense of wholeness and wellness despite his condition.

You can also take these steps to mitigate negative emotions:

- Guide the person in identifying and listing positive coping skills that can help him manage his feelings and behaviors.

- Check in with the person and remind him of his positive coping skills to shift his attention and focus when he feels hopeless, overwhelmed, or powerless.
- If other friends and family members have been the person's confidants in the past, mention it to them and plan activities to get the person out and interacting with others.
- Encourage increased activity and exercise. Endorphins released with exercise help mitigate anxiety and depression. Long walks, massage, or warm baths may relieve anxiety. Take a walk outdoors if weather permits. The outdoors tends to allay anxiety and help the person see the bigger picture when he feels overwhelmed.
- Explore activities the person has enjoyed in the past, or try new activities.
- Encourage adequate sleep. Insomnia can worsen depression.
- Encourage the person to join a support group. Meeting others with a similar condition living a normal life may soothe his anxiety.
- Encourage the person to learn more about heart disease and treatment. Discuss and support him in learning more about heart-related treatment, including diet, medicine, and exercise. People who understand their disease and take control of their care are less depressed and anxious and more hopeful.
- Discourage self-medicating with alcohol, tobacco, or sedatives.

If sad feelings continue, consider talking to the person's doctor or nurse. Beta blockers cause depression or worsen depression in some people. Alternatively, the doctor may consult a psychologist or a psychiatrist to help with the mood disturbance.

I Notice That Since the Last Hospitalization, My Loved One Is Very Angry. Is This Unusual?

Anger leads to the release of adrenaline in the system, which negatively affects blood pressure and may worsen heart failure. It may be a trigger for a heart attack or arrhythmia. It is important to identify irritation, frustration, and anger in people with heart disease and help them learn coping skills to find calm and ease stress.

People with advanced heart disease tend to get angry for many reasons. They may fear the future or be uncertain of how life will unfold. Some feel that no one understands them and that they are alone in their suffering. Others fear a loss of independence and being a burden to others.

Anger is a concern if you notice that the person loses his temper easily or is impatient with others during day-to-day interactions. If he makes disparaging remarks about others' skills, abilities, or trustworthiness, he may have a worrisome anger problem.

How Can I Help the Person Cope with Anger?

Encourage the person to keep a log of his anger, the situations that escalated his anger, and the people he was interacting with at the time. What was his reaction? What other feelings were ongoing at the time of anger? Was there anxiety over another issue?

- Call a time-out. Encourage a break from the current situation or discussion.
- Encourage a mindfulness practice, and participate in it with the person.
- Observe if anxiety is ongoing. If so, follow the recommendations for anxiety listed above.

You can also help the person learn the S.T.O.P. mindfulness method to overcome anger. Remind him to use it at every outburst of anger.

- S is for Stop.
- T is for Take a moment to breathe.
- O is for Observe.
- P is for Proceed to something else.

Talk to the person about how emotions come and go. The emotional response is a ninety-second chemical reaction in the body that then fades away. By not allowing thoughts to linger by ruminating, the emotional response gradually disappears. By revisiting the situation, he will refuel the fire. So you can guide the person to practice the S.T.O.P. method to overcome anger:

- Stop what the person is doing, and get him away from the situation that caused anger.
- Take a few deep breaths. Remind the person to take a minute to breathe normally and naturally, and focus on the breath. Some people concentrate better if they think "breathing in" and "breathing out" while inhaling and exhaling.
- Observe. Have the person observe his experience, including his thoughts, feelings, emotions, posture, pain, and discomfort. The person should reflect on his thoughts and recognize them as such (e.g., "The nurse should

have given me the correct medicine") and observe any emotions about how they are affecting his body (e.g., "I am upset and worried that it will increase my cholesterol"). Observing and naming his emotions will decrease his anger and soothe his mind.

- Proceed. The person should proceed with a supportive action such as talking to a friend, getting a shoulder rub, or drinking a glass of water.

Help the person identify opportunities to practice S.T.O.P. during different occasions. It is not easy, but with practice, it will happen naturally. Ongoing practice will ready the person to use it during triggering situations.

Seven

MEDICATION MANAGEMENT

She used to get confused, miss doses, and then take extra. It was a mess! She was admitted three times because of her confusion with medicine. Everyone was getting frustrated: the doctors, nurses, her, me, everyone. I took charge of filling her pill box, and now it is much better. I have learned so much about medicines in the last six months. Now I feel confident that she is taking the right medicines at the right time.

—*Christopher, whose mother has advanced heart disease*

Modern-day medicines have made the biggest impact on the treatment of heart disease for millions of people around the world. However, incorrect use of medicine is one of the most common causes of harm. Death due to improper use of medicine is not uncommon.

You have a critical role in the person's proper use of medicines to derive benefits without harm. You need to understand what medicines are prescribed, what they are for, when and how to use them, what to do if a dose is missed, what side effects can occur, and what medicine interactions to watch for.

You work with the person to track medicine use. With the help of health care providers, you can understand how medicines must be taken. Make it a weekly routine to help the person set up the pillbox to take the next week. Use daily reminders with an alarm clock or preferably an app on the phone to take the medicines on time.

You should ensure that there is an ample supply of medicines. If any medicines are about to run out, order refills in a timely manner. Maintain a list of medicines, and update it whenever a change is made by any provider. Bring the updated list to each and every clinic visit.

Here is an example of the medicine list that can be used:

Medicine	Dose	Date started	Reason for taking	Side effects/ notes
Metoprolol	25 mg twice a day	12/12/2012	Heart disease	

Also keep a list of discontinued medicines so the doctor is aware of medicines that have been tried in the past:

Medicine	Dose	Date started	Date stopped	Notes
Diltiazem	120 mg once a day	5/6/2006	12/12/2012	Replaced with metoprolol

In women of child-bearing age with heart disease, it is important to consult the cardiologist before embarking on pregnancy since many medicines affect the fetus and later the baby who is breast fed.

This chapter should help people and caregivers understand:

- the role of medicines in the person's condition,
- appropriate use of medicine,
- other medical conditions that may affect the choice of medicines,
- possible interactions between medicines,
- common side effects, and
- other equally effective but cheaper generic alternatives.

This chapter is not a substitute for a doctor's advice but rather a primer to help you work with the doctor in the proper use of medicines.

WHAT MEDICINES ARE USED TO TREAT HEART FAILURE?

The following are the commonly prescribed medicines for people with heart failure:

- beta blockers: halt deterioration of the heart and increase longevity;
- angiotensin-converting enzyme (ACE) inhibitors: control blood pressure, halt deterioration of the heart, and increase longevity;

- angiotensin II receptor blockers: similar to ACE inhibitors;
- diuretics: help eliminate fluid from the body to decrease swelling and shortness of breath;
- spironolactone: improves survival and helps eliminate fluid from the body;
- isosorbide: improves survival and controls angina;
- angiotensin receptor neprilysin inhibitors (ARNI): relax blood vessels, decrease fluid retention, and increase longevity; and
- sodium glucose co-transporter 2 (SGLT2) inhibitors: protect kidneys and increase longevity.

BETA BLOCKERS

Beta blockers are the most commonly used class of heart medicines. Beta blockers' generic and brand names (in parentheses) in the order of use are:

- metoprolol (Lopressor, Toprol-XL),
- atenolol (Tenormin),
- nebivolol (Bystolic),
- bisoprolol (Zebeta),
- propranolol (Inderal LA, InnoPran XL),
- nadolol (Corgard), and
- acebutolol (Sectral).

Although carvedilol (Coreg) may be appropriately considered an alternative to these beta blockers, it belongs to a special class of beta blockers.

Beta blockers are used in many different situations. Often people believe that the doctor has given them this "blood pressure" medicine even though they do not have high blood pressure. In people, beta blockers do more than just decrease blood pressure.

How Do Beta Blockers Work?

Beta blockers block the effect of the adrenaline hormone on the heart. They help the heart function by decreasing heart rate, opening blood vessels, reducing the amount of oxygen heart muscles need to do their work, and lowering blood pressure. Beta blockers prolong life in people after a heart attack. It is not surprising that beta blockers have been the wonder medicines of cardiology for decades.

Uses for Beta Blockers

Doctors prescribe beta blockers for:

- irregular heart rhythms (e.g., atrial fibrillation), to control the heart rate;
- heart failure, to slow the progression of heart failure;
- chest pain (angina), to relieve it;
- heart attacks, to improve long-term survival; and
- high blood pressure, to improve control (usually in addition to other blood pressure medicines).

Beta blockers may also be used to treat overactive thyroid, migraine headaches, and certain kinds of tremors.

What Are the Side Effects?

Beta blockers have been used for decades, and their effects, side effects, and safety have been well studied. Most people who take beta blockers do not have side effects, although some experience:

- fatigue,
- slow heartbeat,
- dizziness or fainting,
- cold hands or feet, or
- weight gain.

Less common side effects include:

- loss of sex drive,
- shortness of breath,
- trouble sleeping, and
- depression.

Tips for Managing Side Effects

Most people get used to the medicine, and the side effects resolve within a few weeks of starting them. However, if they persist, the doctor may suggest one or more of the following steps:

- lowering the dose,
- taking half the dose in the morning and half at night,
- taking the medicine at night, or
- exercising in the morning.

The doctor may also discuss other options. The side effects are reversible (i.e., when the person stops taking the medicine, the side effects resolve).

How to Take the Medicine

Some beta blockers work for twenty-four hours and are taken once a day. Others work for twelve hours and must be taken twice a day. The label on the medicine bottle should explain how much medicine to take and when. The person should take the beta blockers in the morning, at meals, or at bedtime, as instructed on the medicine bottle. These medicines should be taken with food.

How to Stop the Medicine

The person should never stop taking a beta blocker without speaking to the doctor, even if it is not working. Beta blockers need to be tapered from a high to a low dose before stopping completely.

Who Should Avoid Beta Blockers?

People with the following conditions should avoid beta blockers:

- severe asthma,
- fragile diabetes with large fluctuations in blood sugar,
- very slow heart rate, or
- uncontrolled heart failure.

For women who are pregnant or plan to become pregnant, it is critical to discuss the effect of beta blockers on the fetus with the doctor before starting them.

Inform the doctor before starting beta blockers if the person is taking:

- other medicines for high blood pressure;
- medicines for depression;
- medicines for diabetes, including insulin;
- medicines for asthma, chronic bronchitis, emphysema, or chronic obstructive pulmonary disease;
- allergy shots; or
- over-the-counter cough, cold, or allergy medicines.

ANGIOTENSIN-CONVERTING ENZYME (ACE) INHIBITORS

The group of medicines called angiotensin-converting enzyme (ACE) inhibitors have been used for more than three decades. ACE inhibitors by their generic name and then brand name in parentheses in order of use are:

- lisinopril (Prinivil, Zestril),
- enalapril (Vasotec),
- ramipril (Altace),
- benazepril (Lotensin),
- captopril,
- fosinopril,
- moexipril,
- perindopril (Aceon),
- quinapril (Accupril), and
- trandolapril (Mavik).

How Do ACE Inhibitors Work?

ACE is an enzyme that helps produce angiotensin II, a chemical that narrows blood vessels and increases blood pressure. ACE inhibitors block this enzyme to dilate blood vessels and decrease blood pressure, decreasing the heart's workload. In people with a weak heart (cardiomyopathy), ACE inhibitors slow weakening of the heart muscle and increase the life span of many people. ACE inhibitors also slow kidney damage in people with diabetes.

Uses for ACE Inhibitors

ACE inhibitors are used in people with:

- high blood pressure,
- coronary artery disease,
- heart failure, or
- heart attacks.

They are also used in people with diabetes, certain kidney diseases, scleroderma, and migraine.

What Are the Side Effects?

Most people taking ACE inhibitors do not experience side effects. However, some experience:

- a dry, hacking cough;
- fatigue;
- dizziness;
- headaches;
- loss of taste;
- swelling of the face, tongue, throat, legs, or arms (angioedema); or
- increased blood potassium level (hyperkalemia).

A dry cough occurs in one in ten people and may be bothersome enough to switch to a different medicine. In rare cases, people develop swelling of the throat that causes difficulty breathing. This may be life-threatening, and you should call 911 immediately.

Tips for Managing Side Effects

Cough is the most bothersome side effect. In many people, it goes away in a few weeks. In others, decreasing the dose helps resolve the cough. However, if the cough continues to be bothersome, the doctor may switch to a different medicine.

ACE inhibitors can increase potassium levels. The doctor may schedule blood tests to monitor them.

Some people have dizziness or lightheadedness when they start these medicines. The person should stand up slowly from a chair or bed, and you should be there when the person takes the first few doses. If the person faints, call the doctor right away.

In rare cases, a caregiver notices that the person's tongue or lips are swollen and that they are short of breath. In this case, call 911 right away.

How to Take the Medicine

Most ACE inhibitors work for twenty-four hours and should be taken once a day. Rarely, some are taken twice a day. Follow the instructions on the label of the medicine bottle. Older people are typically prescribed lower doses.

The person should take the ACE inhibitor in the morning, one hour before breakfast. If they are taking many medicines that decrease blood pressure, the doctor may advise taking it later in the day.

How to Stop the Medicine

ACE inhibitors decrease the heart's workload and improve heart function. So even if it appears that the ACE inhibitor is not working, the person should not stop taking it without talking to the doctor. People with a heart condition should expect to take this medicine for life.

Who Should Avoid ACE Inhibitors?

Painkillers like ibuprofen (Advil, Motrin) and naproxen (Aleve) interact with ACE inhibitors and decrease their impact. Although occasional use of these painkillers is permitted, if the person takes it on regular basis along with ACE inhibitors, talk to the doctor.

People with a reaction to any previously taken ACE inhibitor should avoid taking other ACE inhibitors.

In combination with salt substitutes, ACE inhibitors may increase the blood potassium level. Talk to the doctor if the person uses salt substitutes; she may either check blood levels more often or switch to another medicine.

In combination with other blood pressure medicines or diuretics, ACE inhibitors can cause a severe drop in blood pressure. However, many people take these medicines together safely.

People taking aliskerin (Tekturna) should not take ACE inhibitors.

ACE inhibitors can cause birth defects. Women who are pregnant or plan to become pregnant should avoid them.

ANGIOTENSIN RECEPTOR BLOCKERS

Several angiotensin receptor blockers (ARBs) are available on the market. Branded and generic versions are available.

ARBs by their generic name and then brand name in parentheses in order of use are:

- valsartan (Diovan),
- losartan (Cozaar),
- irbesartan (Avapro),
- olmesartan (Benicar),
- telmisartan (Micardis),
- azilsartan (Edarbi), and
- candesartan (Atacand).

How Do ARBs Work?

The hormone angiotensin II narrows blood vessels and increases blood pressure. By blocking the action of this hormone, ARBs dilate blood vessels and decrease blood pressure. Lower blood pressure means a lower work-load on the heart. In people with a weak heart (cardiomyopathy), ARBs slow weakening of the heart muscle and increase the life span of many people.

Uses for ARBs

The effects of ARBs are similar to those of ACE inhibitors. ARBs are used as a substitute when ACE inhibitors cause side effects. Similar to ACE inhibitors, ARBs can be used in people with:

- high blood pressure,
- heart failure,
- heart attack, or
- coronary artery disease.

ARBs also protect the kidneys in people with diabetes.

What Are the Side Effects?

Most people taking ARBs do not experience any side effects. However, some have:

- dizziness;
- elevated blood potassium levels (hyperkalemia);
- diarrhea;
- muscle cramps; or
- swelling of the face, tongue, throat, legs, or arms (angioedema).

Some people taking olmesartan experience diarrhea or lose considerable weight. Call the doctor in these situations.

Tips for Managing Side Effects

Like ACE inhibitors, ARBs can increase potassium levels. The doctor monitors the potassium level periodically.

Some people have dizziness or lightheadedness when they start ARBs. You should ensure that the person stands up slowly from beds or chairs. It is important that you are there when the person takes the first few doses. If the person faints, call the doctor immediately.

In rare cases, caregivers may notice swelling of the person's tongue or lips or shortness of breath. If this happens, call 911 right away.

How to Take the Medicine

Most ARBs work for twenty-four hours and should be taken once a day. Follow the instructions on the label of the medicine bottle.

The person may take ARBs on an empty or full stomach in the morning. If the person is taking other medicines that decrease blood pressure, the doctor may recommend taking the ARB later in the day.

How to Stop the Medicine

ARBs keep the blood pressure low, so stopping an ARB suddenly may increase the blood pressure and harm the heart. The person should stop the ARB only under a doctor's supervision.

Who Should Avoid ARBs?

Painkillers like ibuprofen (Advil, Motrin) and naproxen sodium (Aleve) interact with ARBs and decrease their impact. Although occasional use of these painkillers may be acceptable, if the person takes painkillers on a regular basis along with the ARB, talk to the doctor.

Both ARBs and potassium-containing salt substitutes can increase potassium levels in the blood. If the person uses salt substitutes, discuss it with the doctor; she may either check the blood potassium levels more often or switch to another medicine.

If the person has had a reaction to any previously taken ARB, avoid using other ARBs.

People who use other blood pressure medicines or diuretics may have a severe drop in blood pressure and should be cautious. However, many people take more than one blood pressure medicine safely.

You should discuss it with the doctor if the person takes any of these medicines:

- the aliskiren group of medicines (Tekturna, Tekamlo, Amturnide);
- lithium (Lithobid);
- digoxin (specifically with telmisartan); or
- warfarin (specifically with telmisartan).

In general, ARBs and ACE inhibitors should not be used together because they have similar effects.

ARBs can harm a developing fetus. Women who are pregnant or plan to become pregnant should avoid them.

DIURETICS

Diuretics, or water pills, have been used in one form or another for centuries. Generic and brand-name diuretics are available on the market:

- hydrochlorothiazide (Microzide),
- furosemide (Lasix),
- spironolactone (Aldactone),
- chlorothiazide (Diuril),
- bumetanide (Bumex),
- chlorthalidone,
- metolazone,
- torsemide (Demadex),
- indapamide,
- ethacrynic acid (Edecrin),
- amiloride,
- eplerenone (Inspra), and
- triamterene (Dyrenium).

Diuretics are often used in combination with other blood pressure medicines.

How Do Diuretics Work?

Diuretics help the kidneys excrete more salt and water as urine so less fluid is in blood vessels, reducing blood pressure.

What Are the Uses for Diuretics?

Diuretics have been used to control blood pressure for decades. Diuretics help when fluid retention is a problem in people with heart failure, liver failure, and certain kidney problems.

What Are the Side Effects?

Diuretics are generally safe, and most people do not have any side effects. However, with increased urination, electrolytes and minerals are lost. People need to be monitored for blood levels of sodium, calcium, and magnesium. Some people have low blood pressure and dizziness as a result of fluid loss. Increased blood sugar, gout attacks, headaches, dehydration, and muscle cramps are other side effects.

Tips for Managing Side Effects

If frequent bathroom visits bother the person at night, talk to the doctor about changing the timing of the diuretics. The person will have periodic blood tests to monitor electrolytes and minerals.

How to Take the Medicine

Different diuretics remain in the body for different times. Depending on the situation, the doctor may prescribe the medicine to be taken one or more times a day. The label on the medicine bottle should tell you how much and how often the person should take the medicine.

The person should take the diuretic early in the day. The second dose, if prescribed, should be taken by mid-afternoon to avoid frequent bathroom visits at night.

How to Stop the Medicine

Like all blood pressure–lowering medicine, most people remain on diuretics for life, although the doctor may change the dose and/or frequency. A change in the dose may require a simultaneous change in potassium supplement intake. The person should not change or stop the medicine without talking to the doctor.

Who Should Avoid or Be Cautious with Diuretics?

The following conditions put people at risk for side effects:

- gout,
- kidney stones,
- liver or kidney problems,
- frequent episodes of dehydration and dizziness,
- allergy to sulfa medicines, and
- pregnancy.

Drug Interactions

Diuretics interact with other medicines and supplements, such as:

- other blood pressure medicines;
- antidepressants such as fluoxetine (Prozac) and venlafaxine (Effexor XR);
- herbal medicines or supplements such as hawthorn, parsley, and green and black tea;

- lithium; and
- cyclosporine (Restasis).

Any Other Precautions with Using Diuretics?

Ongoing diuretic use may require routine blood tests. You should ensure that the person does not get dehydrated. Depending on the diuretic, the doctor may prescribe a potassium supplement.

STATINS

What Are Statins?

Statins, a group of medicines that lower cholesterol levels, have been used for more than three decades. Available generic and brand-name statins are:

- atorvastatin (Lipitor),
- simvastatin (Zocor),
- rosuvastatin (Crestor),
- pravastatin (Pravachol),
- fluvastatin (Lescol),
- cerivastatin (Baychol),
- lovastatin (Altoprev),
- pitavastatin (Livalo), and
- mevastatin.

Combination medicines containing a statin (e.g., Vytorin, with simvastatin) are also available.

How Do Statins Work?

An enzyme in the liver, HMG CoA reductase, controls the production of cholesterol. Statins block this enzyme, slowing the production of cholesterol to decrease its level in the blood. Statins also decrease inflammation, stabilize the lining of coronary blood vessels, and decrease the risk of heart attack.

Who Should Take Statins?

Statins are prescribed to people who have high cholesterol or are at high risk for heart disease. In people with heart disease or stroke, statins decrease the risk of heart attack and prolong life.

What Are the Side Effects?

Most people do not have side effects from statins. However, one-third have muscle pain, soreness, or weakness. Rarely, this affects the person's daily activities or causes life-threatening muscle damage called rhabdomyolysis, which causes severe muscle pain, liver damage, kidney failure, and death. Other side effects include:

- minor increases in liver enzymes;
- rarely, liver damage causing unusual fatigue and weakness, yellow eyes or skin, dark urine, pain in the abdomen, and loss of appetite;
- increased blood sugar; and
- memory loss or confusion.

Other minor side effects include a rash, headache, abdominal pain, bloating, diarrhea, and a tingling sensation (i.e., "pins and needles") in the arms and legs.

Tips for Managing Side Effects

Millions of people worldwide use statins without side effects. However, some do develop some of the side effects mentioned previously. Consult the doctor to find an appropriate solution for statin-related side effects.

For liver problems, the person should have a liver enzyme test before and after starting a statin. Watch for signs of liver damage (e.g., unusual fatigue and weakness, yellow eyes or skin, dark urine, abdominal pain, loss of appetite).

One-third of people taking statins have muscle pain. Here are options to consider in consultation with the doctor:

- Stop the statin for a few days and see if the muscle pain goes away. This will help determine if the muscle pain is indeed related to the statin.
- Decrease the dose of statin or change to another statin.
- Use another cholesterol-lowering medicine.
- Refrain from vigorous exercise.

How to Take the Medicine

Statins are taken once a day. Some people take their statin in the morning, while others take theirs at night. Follow the instructions on the label of the medicine bottle. Some brands should be taken with food, while others may be taken with or without it. Ask the pharmacist when the person should take the statin.

Most people continue to use statins their whole life to keep cholesterol low and protect them against heart disease and stroke.

How to Stop the Medicine

Most people take statins their whole life, but in people with side effects, doctors may lower the dose or switch to another statin or a non-statin cholesterol-lowering medicine. Consult the doctor before the person stops a statin.

Who Should Avoid Statins?

These people are likely to have side effects from statins and should be cautious:

- women who are pregnant or planning to become pregnant,
- those age sixty-five years or older,
- those with small body size,
- those taking multiple medicines for cholesterol,
- those with excessive alcohol use, and
- those with liver or kidney problems.

Statins interact with many medicines, such as:

- diltiazem (Cartia, Dilacor XR, Diltzac, Taztia, Tiazac);
- verapamil (Calan, Isoptin);
- fenofibrate (Antara, Fenoglide, Lipofen, Lofibra, TriCor, Triglide);
- gemfibrozil (Lopid), another kind of cholesterol-lowering medicine;
- erythromycin;
- itraconazole (Onmel, Sporanox);
- clarithromycin (Biaxin);
- amiodarone (Cordarone, Pacerone), a heart rhythm medicine;
- some immunosuppressant medicines (e.g., cyclosporine [Gengraf, Neoral, Sandimmune]);
- protease inhibitors;
- amprenavir (Agenerase);
- atazanavir (Reyataz);
- darunavir (Prezista);
- fosamprenavir (Telzir, Lexiva);

- indinavir (Crixivan);
- lopinavir/ritonavir (Kaletra, Aluvia);
- nelfinavir (Viracept);
- ritonavir (Norvir);
- saquinavir (Invirase); and
- tipranavir (Aptivus).

WARFARIN

Warfarin, a blood thinner used in people to prevent stroke, has been in medical use since 1954. It is sold under the brand names Coumadin and Jantoven.

How Does Warfarin Work?

Vitamin K is required to produce chemicals that help blood clot. Warfarin blocks the action of Vitamin K, decreasing clotting of the blood.

Uses for Warfarin

Warfarin is used in people with atrial fibrillation or artificial metallic valves. Rarely, it is prescribed when people have blood clots in the heart. It is also used in non-cardiac conditions to prevent and treat deep venous thrombosis and pulmonary embolism.

Newer medicines such as dabigatran (Pradaxa), apixaban (Eliquis), edoxaban (Savaysa), and rivaroxaban (Xarelto) offer the efficacy of warfarin without the need for monitoring.

Like warfarin, aspirin falls into the category of "blood thinner." However, the two are not equivalent and cannot be used interchangeably. Clopidogrel (Plavix), prasugrel (Effient), and ticagrelor (Brilinta) also have specific uses and are not equivalents of warfarin.

What Are the Side Effects?

Bleeding is the most common side effect of warfarin. Minor bruises are common. Bleeding gums, blood-tinged urine, blood while blowing the nose in the morning, excessive bruising, and minor increases in menstrual flow are not uncommon. In rare cases, people develop life-threatening bleeding (e.g., in the gastrointestinal system or brain). People with no other risk factors for bleeding have about a 1 percent risk of major bleeding due to warfarin. In people with other risk factors for bleeding, this risk goes up substantially. It is important to talk with the doctor about the risk of bleeding when she prescribes warfarin.

Another concern with warfarin is skin necrosis, or gangrene. If the person has pain, a color change or warmth in any area of the body, or pain and purple discoloration in the toes, call the doctor immediately.

Some people report a "pins and needles" sensation in the arms or legs, thinning of the hair, bloating, flatulence, and an unusual or bad taste in the mouth.

How to Take the Medicine

When a person is prescribed warfarin, he is enrolled in a "warfarin clinic" or "Coumadin clinic." This is generally a pharmacist-run clinic that checks the effects of warfarin on the blood. This is generally measured as the international normalized ratio (INR) (e.g., INR 1.7 or 2.5). The doctor decides the target range of INR according to the person's health condition. If the INR is low, the clinic increases the prescribed dose. If it is higher than the target range, the dose is lowered.

This clinic is the best place to ask questions about food to avoid with the use of warfarin. Typically, the person should eat food rich in vitamin K in similar portions week after week. Large fluctuations in the use of these food items cause fluctuations in INR levels, which is dangerous. The specific food items are asparagus, broccoli, Brussels sprouts, cabbage, green leafy vegetables (e.g., collards, turnip greens, mustard greens, spinach, salad greens), plums, and rhubarb. Soybean and canola oil also fall into this category.

The person may be advised to vary the doses of warfarin every day. Follow the warfarin clinic's instructions. Do not use more or less of it. These tablets can be taken on a full or empty stomach.

Grapefruit juice interacts with warfarin. If the person drinks grapefruit juice, talk to the warfarin clinic.

If there is minor bleeding while on warfarin, the doctor may continue warfarin because the benefit is more than the risk. However, if there is a life-threatening bleed with the need for a blood transfusion, the doctor may stop warfarin and start a different medicine. Alternatively, she may discuss other options and stop blood thinners altogether. However, this has to be done after a thorough discussion and understanding of the risks and benefits of the options.

Dosing

The correct dose of warfarin varies from person to person. Depending on how the person's body reacts to warfarin, the warfarin clinic may alter the dose so as to get the INR into the required range. The person may be asked to take a different dose on different days of the week. Follow the warfarin clinic's instructions.

Missed Doses

If the person misses a dose of warfarin, he should take it as soon as possible. However, if it is almost time for the next dose, skip the missed dose and resume the regular schedule. Do not double doses.

How to Stop the Medicine

A doctor may stop Warfarin temporarily (e.g., before surgery) or permanently (due to side effects or in favor of an alternative medicine). Remember that the effect of warfarin lasts for three days after it is stopped.

Warfarin and Surgery

Special precaution is needed when people taking warfarin need surgery. Typically, the surgeon asks permission from the cardiologist to stop it for five days. Depending on the situation, the cardiologist may agree to stop warfarin and restart it after a few days. Alternatively, she may request a temporary switch to other blood thinners to prevent blood clots and stroke.

Who Should Avoid Warfarin?

Warfarin is notorious for interacting with other medicines. A useful list of such medicines is available at depts.washington.edu/anticoag/home/content/warfarin-medicine-interactions.

Warfarin also interacts with foods such as avocados, black and green tea, soybeans, and foods rich in vitamin K.

Because warfarin decreases the blood's ability to clot, it must be avoided or used with caution in people with certain other conditions:

- anemia;
- frequent falls;
- uncontrolled high blood pressure;
- kidney disease;

- liver damage;
- use of other blood thinners;
- blood disorders (e.g., polycythemia vera, protein C deficiency, thrombocytopenia);
- previous or active gastric or intestinal ulcer;
- previous or active bleeding problems;
- vasculitis (inflammation of the blood vessels);
- previous brain surgery;
- previous bleeding in the brain;
- aneurysm in the brain; or
- excessive alcohol use.

Women who are pregnant or who plan to become pregnant should not use warfarin.

AMIODARONE

Amiodarone has been used for more than half a century. It is an antiarrhythmic, a medicine used to treat abnormal heart rhythms. It is one of the most effective medicines in its class. Amiodarone is sold under the brand names Cordarone and Pacerone.

How Does Amiodarone Work?

Amiodarone is a multipurpose antiarrhythmic medicine with multiple effects on the heart's electrical system. It primarily affects the potassium channel in the heart tissue to prevent abnormal rhythms.

Uses for Amiodarone

Doctors prescribe amiodarone to help manage rhythm problems affecting the upper chamber (atrial fibrillation) or lower chamber (ventricular tachycardia or fibrillation) of the heart.

What Are the Side Effects?

Amiodarone is notorious for causing multiple side effects. One may notice minor, transient side effects such as headache, loss of appetite, nausea, vomiting, dizziness, and fatigue. The following are concerning side effects that appear after taking amiodarone for months or years:

- lung problems such as cough, fever, shortness of breath, or difficulty breathing;
- eye problems such as blurred vision, increased sensitivity to light, and dry eye;
- liver problems (rare) such as yellowing of the skin or eyes or loss of appetite;
- thyroid problems such as dry, puffy skin; increased sensitivity to heat or cold; or unusual fatigue; and
- tingling or numbness in hands or feet, hand tremors, or weakness in the arms or legs.

Tips for Managing Side Effects

The person should get these tests regularly to look for side effects from amiodarone:

- electrocardiogram,
- blood test to assess liver function,
- blood test to assess thyroid function,
- regular eye exams, and
- chest radiograph and lung function test.

Amiodarone increases sensitivity to sunlight, so the person should stay out of sunlight when possible and wear a hat and sunglasses and use sunscreen when exposed to the sun. The person should not use a tanning bed while taking amiodarone.

Grapefruit can increase the amount of amiodarone in the body and thus the chances of side effects. Talk to the doctor before including grapefruit juice as a part of the person's regular diet.

How to Take the Medicine

Amiodarone takes weeks to build up in the body. Often, the person is asked to start with a large dose of amiodarone and taper it over weeks (e.g., start with 400 mg tablets three times a day for a two weeks, then 400 mg tablets two times a day for two weeks, then 400 mg tablets once a day for two weeks, and then 200 mg tablets once a day). The doses may vary depending on the person's condition. Follow the instructions from the doctor, nurse, or pharmacist. In some cases, amiodarone is given intravenously in the hospital and then a regular dose is chosen at release from the hospital.

If the person accidentally misses a dose of amiodarone, the person should take the missed dose within two or three hours. If it is almost time for the next dose, the person should skip the missed dose and resume the regular schedule. The person should not take two doses at the same time. Amiodarone should be taken with food.

How to Stop the Medicine

In some cases, the doctor may prescribe amiodarone for a short time and then discontinue it. Or she may continue it for a longer time and stop it when it is no longer effective.

Amiodarone may be stopped under the guidance of a doctor when it is no longer effective or the person develops side effects from it. It does not need to be tapered.

Amiodarone remains in the body for a long time, so its effects continue for weeks after stopping it. It is important to let the doctors know if amiodarone was recently stopped.

Who Should Avoid Amiodarone?

Amiodarone has a number of long-term side effects, so it should be avoided in young people who may need rhythm-related medicine for a number of years. People of advanced age may be prescribed a lower dose of amiodarone.

Caution is required in the use of amiodarone in people with:

- slow heartbeats,
- preexisting eye problems,
- low potassium or magnesium,
- preexisting lung conditions,
- preexisting thyroid conditions, or
- preexisting liver disease.

Amiodarone interacts with many medicines, including warfarin and digoxin. Dose adjustment may be required when they are taken together. A list of other medicines that interact with amiodarone is provided at medicines .com/medicine-interactions/amiodarone.html.

Amiodarone is typically avoided in women who are pregnant or plan to become pregnant.

Amiodarone produces electrocardiogram changes. Adding other medicines, herbs, or supplements may worsen this situation and cause side effects. It is very important to talk to the doctor before the person starts a new prescription or over-the-counter medicine.

ANTIPLATELET MEDICINES

Aspirin, an antiplatelet medicine, has been used for more than a century. Newer antiplatelet medicines such as clopidogrel (1997), prasugrel (2009), and ticagrelor (2011) are also on the market.

Aspirin is the most commonly used antiplatelet medicine. However, it is a very important, special medicine that will be discussed separately. Here, we will restrict our discussion to other common antiplatelet medicines:

- clopidogrel (Plavix),
- prasugrel (Effient), and
- ticagrelor (Brilinta).

Other medicines on the market (but not commonly used) are:

- ticlopidine (Ticlid) and
- dipyridamole (Aggrenox).

Some medicines in this group are available in generic and brand-name options, while others are not available in generic form (e.g., Brilinta).

How Do Antiplatelet Medicines Work?

In response to injury, platelets become active and clump together. These platelets release chemicals to start a series of reactions and form a protein called fibrin, which attaches to the platelet clump to form a blood clot.

Clots form in response to injury to prevent excessive bleeding. However, if the platelets react and start the formation of clots in an artery when there is no bleeding, they block the vessel. If this happens in a coronary artery, it can cause a heart attack. If it happens in a blood vessel in the brain, it can cause a stroke.

Antiplatelet medicines work by preventing activation of the platelets, the first step in clot formation. By preventing clot formation, they can help prevent heart attacks and strokes.

Uses for Antiplatelet Medicines

Antiplatelet medicines are commonly used in people with:

- previous heart attack,
- peripheral vascular disease,
- previous stroke, or
- stent placement.

These antiplatelet agents may or may not be interchangeable, depending on the condition being treated. Doctors may choose a specific one according to the person's medical condition.

What Are the Side Effects?

Although most people using antiplatelet medicines do not have side effects, some do, especially when starting the medicine.

By preventing blood clots, antiplatelet medicines may increase bleeding. It may be minor (e.g., nose bleed, easy bruising, heavy bleeding from minor cuts, unusually heavy menstrual bleeding). However, if the person coughs up blood, has black tarry stools, or vomits coffee-ground-like liquid, it can be dangerous. Call 911 in such cases.

Other side effects include gastrointestinal upset (e.g., nausea, stomach pain, diarrhea). A rash and itching may be noted in some cases.

In rare situations, people develop wheezing, difficulty breathing, tightness in the chest, fever, chills, sore throat, swelling of the face or hands, or ringing in the ears after starting these medicines. These side effects can be worse in people with asthma and allergies. These conditions require immediate attention.

If you notice fever and confusion, it may indicate a very rare but dangerous side effect called thrombotic thrombocytopenic purpura (TTP), for which immediate medical attention is needed. People using ticlopidine have a much higher risk of this than people taking other antiplatelet medicines. Ticlopidine is also associated with other blood conditions, including low white cell count (neutropenia) and a decrease in all blood cell count (aplastic anemia).

Tips for Managing Side Effects

Minor bruising, nose bleeds, or blood-tinged urine may occur initially. These side effects may be bothersome, but in most people the benefit of antiplatelet medicine is higher than these minor risks. However, in case of excessive bleeding, the doctor may consider switching the medicine, stopping other medicines that may be interacting with the antiplatelet medicine, or even stopping the antiplatelet medicine.

The risk of TTP and other blood disorders with ticlopidine is highest during the first three months of taking the medicine. Thus, it is critical for the person to see the doctor and get lab tests to monitor for these possible side effects.

How to Take the Medicine

Most antiplatelet medicines are taken once or twice a day. They should not be taken on an empty stomach. These medicines may be prescribed for one month, six months, one year, or life, depending on the person's condition.

Missed Doses

The person should take the missed dose if it is recognized within a couple of hours. However, if it has been several hours, he should skip the missed dose and resume the regular dosing schedule. Do not double doses. Taking higher doses or more frequent doses of antiplatelet medicines increases the risk of serious side effects.

How to Stop the Medicine

If the person has had a stent placed, antiplatelet medicines should not be stopped unless directed by the doctor. People who stop them even for a day run a large risk of their stent getting clogged, leading to a heart attack. Therefore, it is important to have enough of a supply and take the medicine regularly. Do not run out of this medicine; plan ahead and call for refills.

Before any surgery, dental procedure, or emergency treatment, tell the doctor or dentist that the person is taking this medicine. They may seek the cardiologist's permission to stop the antiplatelet medicines for five to seven days.

Who Should Avoid Antiplatelet Medicines?

Because antiplatelet medicines increase the risk of bleeding, they should be used with caution in people with:

- previous bleeding due to peptic ulcer,
- previous bleeding in the head,

- severe liver disease,
- blood disorders that cause increased bleeding, or
- a prescription for another blood thinner (e.g., warfarin).

People allergic to aspirin, ibuprofen, or naproxen should mention this to their doctor when she suggests antiplatelet medicines.

Antiplatelet medicines interact with some medicines:

- antacids,
- digoxin,
- defibrotide,
- fluvastatin,
- itraconazole,
- non-steroidal anti-inflammatory medicines (e.g., aspirin, ibuprofen, naproxen),
- oseltamivir (Tamiflu),
- simvastatin (Zocor),
- tamoxifen,
- theophylline,
- warfarin, and
- herbal or natural supplements.

The doctor may choose a lower dose or monitor closely for medicine interactions if she knows that the person is taking these medicines.

Aggrenox interacts with ACE inhibitors, beta blockers, and diuretics to decrease the effects of those medicines. The doctor may choose to monitor closely or change the dose of medicine to counter this interaction.

ISOSORBIDE

Isosorbide has been used since 1981. A long-acting version of nitroglycerin, it is available as isosorbide dinitrate (Isordil) and isosorbide mononitrate (Imdur, Imdur ER, Ismo, Monoket). It prevents chest pain in people with coronary artery disease and is available in both generic and brand-name forms.

How Does Isosorbide Work?

Isosorbide relaxes and widens all arteries, including the coronary arteries, and increases blood and oxygen flow to the heart while decreasing the heart's workload. Thus, it increases the oxygen supply to the heart and decreases oxygen demand from the heart. This prevents angina, or chest pain, when the medicine is used regularly on a long-term basis.

Uses for Isosorbide

Isosorbide is used to prevent chest pain in people with coronary artery disease. It is also used in African Americans with heart failure. Some people with esophageal spasm also benefit from it.

What Are the Side Effects?

Isosorbide causes headache in most people, which indicates that it is working. Because it decreases blood pressure, people may feel lightheaded or dizzy if they stand up suddenly. Alcohol use, dehydration, hot weather, and vigorous exercise may further decrease blood pressure and cause dizziness or fainting. Other side effects include blurred vision, fatigue, sleep disturbances, and gastrointestinal upset.

How to Manage the Side Effects

A headache indicates that the medicine is potent and working. People should not stop using the medicine or change its dose or timing. If the pain is severe and intolerable, talk to the doctor.

To avoid dizziness and lightheadedness when rising from a lying or sitting position, the person should drink lots of water and avoid alcohol and hot weather. Getting up slowly and stabilizing before walking helps.

How to Take the Medicine

Isosorbide mononitrate is taken once a day in the morning. Isosorbide dinitrate is taken twice a day, first in the morning and then six or seven hours later. The doctor may increase the dose if it does not have the desired effect.

Both these medicines are slowly released into the blood over hours, so they do not provide instant relief from chest pain like nitroglycerin. The person should use short-acting nitroglycerin if he has chest pain despite the use of isosorbide.

The extended-release form of isosorbide should not be split or crushed; rather, it should be swallowed whole.

If the person misses a dose, he can take it within an hour or two of the missed dose. If it is almost time for the next dose, skip the missed dose and resume the regular schedule. Do not double the dose because it may drop the blood pressure to a dangerous level.

How to Stop the Medicine

The person should not stop using isosorbide without checking with the doctor, who may advise a slow taper of the medicine.

Who Should Avoid Isosorbide?

Because this medicine can decrease blood pressure, people with these conditions should be cautious when starting isosorbide:

- low blood pressure,
- tendency toward frequent dehydration, and
- hypertrophic cardiomyopathy.

If the person is allergic to nitrates (e.g., amyl nitrate, butyl nitrate) or nitrites, avoid isosorbide.

The following medicines, when used with isosorbide, cause a sudden and dangerous drop in blood pressure:

- avanafil,
- riociguat,
- sildenafil,
- tadalafil, and
- vardenafil.

The doctor may change the medicine or not start isosorbide in people taking these medicines.

A combination of isosorbide and calcium channel blockers (e.g., diltiazem, cardizem) may lead to a significant decrease in blood pressure. Propranolol also may interact with isosorbide, especially in people with severe liver damage.

SOTALOL

Sotalol, like amiodarone, is an antiarrhythmic medicine used to control the heart rhythm. Sotalol has been used since 1974 and is available in both generic and brand-name forms:

- Betapace,
- Betapace AF,
- Sorine, and
- Sotylize.

How Does Sotalol Work?

Sotalol belongs to two different classes of medicine that prevent abnormal rhythms and maintain normal ones:

- Beta blocker (e.g., metoprolol, atenolol): It blocks the effect of the hormone adrenaline on the beta receptors in the heart muscle.
- Potassium channel-blocking antiarrhythmic medicine (e.g., amiodarone): It affects the electrical conduction system of the heart through the potassium channel in the heart tissue.

Uses for Sotalol

As an antiarrhythmic medicine, sotalol is used to control atrial arrhythmias (e.g., atrial fibrillation) and ventricular arrhythmias (e.g., ventricular tachycardia, ventricular fibrillation, premature ventricular contractions).

What Are the Side Effects?

Sotalol is a potassium channel-blocking medicine, so it has specific effects on the potassium channels in the heart cells. In the right amount, it controls the heart rhythm and is beneficial. However, if the heart cells are exposed to large amounts, a dangerous rhythm called torsades de pointes can occur. Frequent electrocardiograms determine if too much sotalol is in the body.

Some doctors prefer to start this medicine in the hospital, where they can monitor the electrocardiography regularly and adjust the dose.

Sotalol slows the heart, like other beta blockers, which may result in fatigue, dizziness, lightheadedness, confusion, and blurred vision. In some patients it may cause exacerbation of asthma.

Tips for Managing Side Effects

Sotalol can cause dangerous arrhythmias if there is too much in the blood. By monitoring regular electrocardiography, the doctor can ensure safe levels of sotalol.

Sotalol interacts with many other medicines, so tell the doctor that the person is taking sotalol when any new medicine is prescribed. This website has a list of medicines that may interact with sotalol: medicines.com/medicine-interactions/sotalol.html.

Fatigue, though bothersome in the beginning, may improve over time. Fainting, lightheadedness, and dizziness may be related to a low heart rate caused by sotalol. It is important to monitor the heart rate and pulse when starting sotalol. If the heart rate is lower than 50 beats per minute during the day, tell the doctor, who may change the dose or recommend alternatives.

How to Take the Medicine

Once the doctor has determined the right dose based on electrocardiography, the person should take it as prescribed. Most people take this medicine twice a day, twelve hours apart. Changing the dose or frequency of use leads to dangerous side effects.

Do not run out of this medicine; plan to call and get refills. The person should not take this medicine within two hours of taking antacids. Stick to either the generic or brand name because switching back and forth is not advisable.

After a missed dose, the person can take it within two or three hours. However, if it is almost time for the next dose, skip the missed dose and resume the regular schedule. Under no circumstances should you double the dose to make up for the missed one.

How to Stop the Medicine

Sotalol should be stopped only under the guidance of a doctor, even if it is not working or is causing side effects. She may choose to taper the dose before stopping it completely.

Who Should Avoid Sotalol?

People with these problems should avoid or be cautious with sotalol:
- kidney problems;
- slow heart rate;
- heart pumping (ejection fraction) less than 40 percent (normal, 55 percent);
- asthma;
- prolonged QT segment on electrocardiography;

- previous problems with other beta blockers; or
- trouble with electrolyte balance.

Many medicines interact with sotalol. A complete list of them is available at medicines.com/medicine-interactions/sotalol.html. Before the person starts a new medicine while taking sotalol, check this website to ensure its safety when taken with sotalol.

Most doctors avoid this medicine in pregnant and breastfeeding women.

ASPIRIN

An early form of aspirin found in the leaves of willow trees was known for its health effects and used for more than two millennia. The current form, acetylsalicylic acid, was produced in 1853, and Bayer has marketed it under the name "aspirin" since 1899.

In addition to the generic form, it is sold under these brand names:

- Ascriptin,
- Aspergum,
- Aspirtab,
- Bayer,
- Easprin,
- Ecotrin,
- Ecpirin,
- Entercote,
- Genacote,
- Halfprin,
- Ninoprin, and
- Norwich Aspirin.

How Does Aspirin Work?

Aspirin, like other antiplatelet medicines, prevents clot formation by interfering with platelet clumping. It also works as a painkiller and anti-fever medicine.

Uses for Aspirin

Aspirin is a common heart medicine used to lower the risk of heart attack in people and risk of recurrent stroke in people who had an ischemic stroke or transient ischemic attack.

Although it is a "blood thinner," it is not a good replacement for warfarin in people who are recommended warfarin for atrial fibrillation. Likewise, it is not a good replacement for clopdiogrel, prasugrel, or ticagrelor after stent placement.

What Are the Side Effects?

Most people tolerate aspirin without any side effects. The most common side effect is inflammation of the esophagus and stomach, resulting in heartburn. This condition is aggravated by the use of alcohol, tobacco, and medicines such as ibuprofen and naproxen.

Also, blood thinners such as warfarin, Eliquis, Pradxa, and Xarelto increase the risk of bleeding from an inflamed stomach and esophagus. Such bleeding is noted as black tarry stools or vomiting blood or liquid that looks like coffee grounds. In rare cases, aspirin causes hives and swelling.

Tips for Managing Side Effects

In some cases, decreasing the dose may relieve some side effects of aspirin. Enteric-coated aspirin may prevent inflammation of the esophagus and stomach. Using medicines to protect against gastritis may help the person tolerate aspirin.

How to Take the Medicine

The dose of aspirin depends on the condition for which it is used. Thus, it is important to take it as prescribed.

If the aspirin is in the capsule or extended-release form, the person should swallow it whole and avoid crushing, breaking, or chewing it. If a dose was missed within two or three hours, the person should take the dose of aspirin. If it has been longer, skip the missed dose.

How to Stop the Medicine

In some people, aspirin may be prescribed lifelong. Before surgery, the surgeon may stop aspirin for five to seven days. It is not necessary to taper the aspirin dose.

Who Should Avoid Aspirin?

There are certain people for whom aspirin may do more harm than good, such as those with:

- an allergy to ibuprofen, naproxen, or other painkillers;
- asthma with nasal polyps and rhinitis;
- reflux disease;
- peptic ulcer disease or bleeding related to ulcers;
- severe kidney disease;
- severe liver disease;
- the rare blood disorder hemolytic anemia; or
- gout.

Aspirin interacts with these medicines and decreases their effects:

- the diabetes medicines tolbutamide and chlorpropamide,
- warfarin,
- methotrexate,
- the epilepsy medicines phenytoin and valproic acid,
- probenecid,
- steroids, and
- spironolactone.

Aspirin should not be used in the later stages of pregnancy.

ANGIOTENSIN RECEPTOR NEPRILYSIN INHIBITORS (ARNI)

ARNI are a new class of medicines used in patients with heart failure. The currently available ARNI is sacubitril/vasartan, which is sold under the brand name of Entresto.

ARNI are used in patients who have heart failure from decreased pumping function of the heart.

How Do ARNI Work?

ARNI block the effect of neprilysin and angiotension II and hence help relax the blood vessels and open them up. This in turn makes sure the body does not retain fluid and hence improves symptoms of heart failure.

ARNI have been shown to improve longevity and decrease hospitalization in patients with heart failure.

Uses for ARNI

Doctors prescribe ARNI for patients with weak pumping of the heart resulting in heart failure.

What Are the Side Effects?

ARNI are a new class of medicines, but some of the side effects are known such as:

- low blood pressure causing dizziness and lightheadedness (this is especially worrisome in older patients over seventy-five years of age);
- swelling of the face, throat, tongue, legs, or arms (angioedema);
- diarrhea;
- headache;
- gastritis; and
- worsening renal function.

Less common side effects include:

- cough,
- decrease in red blood cell count,
- fatigue,
- nausea, and
- low level of blood sugar.

Tips for Managing Side Effects

If you have swelling of the throat, face, tongue, arms, or legs or have difficulty swallowing after taking the first dose, call 911 immediately.

Most people taking ARNI do not experience any side effects. However, if you do experience any side effects, talk to your doctor. She may review your medical history and other medications and suggest lowering the dose if needed.

How to Take the Medicine

It is important to stop ACEI two days before starting ARNI. Generally patients are started on a low dose, and the dose is gradually increased under physician supervision. ARNI should be taken twice a day, once in the morning and once in the evening, with or without food. The medicine should be taken about the same time every day. The physician will routinely review blood pressure and kidney functions while the person is taking ARNI.

On a given day, if the person forgets to take a dose, take it as soon as it is remembered. However, if it is almost time for the next dose, skip the missed dose. Do not take a double dose to make up for the missed dose.

How to Stop the Medicine

The person should never stop taking ARNI without speaking to the doctor, even if you feel that it is not working.

Who Should Avoid ARNI?

People with the following conditions should avoid ARNI:

- low blood pressure (systolic BP below100mm Hg),
- intolerance of ACEI or ARB,
- high levels of potassium,
- significant kidney problems,
- significant liver problem,
- very severe heart failure causing shortness of breath at rest,
- pregnant women and those anticipating getting pregnant, and
- women who are breast feeding or plan to breast feed.

Inform the doctor before starting ARNI if the person is taking:

- ACEI;
- statins;
- potassium supplements;
- spironolactone;
- NSAIDs such as ibuprofen, naproxen, etc.;
- sildenafil;
- Lasix;
- metformin for diabetes;
- lithium; or
- aliskerin.

SODIUM-GLUCOSE TRANSPORT PROTEIN 2 (SGLT2) INHIBITORS

SGLT2 inhibitors, also known as gliflozins, are a new class of medicines for patients with heart failure, especially those who also have diabetes. Since they are new medicines, information on these medicines is evolving.

Pharmaceutical and brand names of the various SGLT2 inhibitors available on the market are:

- dapagliflozin (Farxiga),
- canagliflozin (Invokana),
- empagliflozin (Jardiance), and
- ertugliflozin (Steglatro).

In heart patients, dapagliflozin and empagliflozin are most commonly used.

How Do the SGLT2 Inhibitors Work?

SGLT2 inhibitors promote loss of glucose through the urine and hence help diabetic patients achieve good glucose control. In diabetic patients who have weak pumping of the heart, it promotes fluid loss and hence improves symptoms of heart failure. Recent research shows that it helps in non-diabetic patients also. Overall, patients with weak pumping function of the heart taking SGLT2 inhibitors have increased longevity and decreased hospitalization.

Uses for SGLT2 Inhibitors

SGLT2 inhibitors are used in patients with weak pumping of the heart. They are especially helpful in patients with diabetes. Please note that SGLT2 inhibitors are also prescribed for diabetics who may not have heart problems since these medicines improve glucose control and protect the kidneys in diabetic patients.

What Are the Side Effects?

Common side effects of SGLT2 inhibitors include:

- low blood pressure, which causes lightheadedness and dizziness;
- low blood sugar;
- increased urinary tract infection;
- increased chance of yeast infection;
- diabetic ketoacidosis (dangerously high levels of blood sugar) with symptoms of nausea, abdominal pain, unusual amount of thirst, difficulty breathing, confusion, or unusual fatigue; and
- increased cholesterol.

Minor side effects include:

- nausea,
- constipation,
- back pain,
- joint pain,
- nasal congestion and flu-like symptoms, and
- increased thirst.

Rare but serious side effects with SGLT2 inhibitors include:

- genital infection with symptoms of pain, redness, or swelling in the genital area; fever; or malaise;
- increased risk of limb amputation;
- bone fracture; and
- kidney failure.

Tips for Managing Side Effects

SGLT2 inhibitors may cause loss of fluid and dehydration. It is important to start the medicine under strict supervision and inform the doctor if the person notices increased urination along with increased thirst, lightheadedness, and dizziness. While taking these medicines, it is important to assess blood sugar and kidney functions regularly.

How to Take the Medicine

The doctor will check kidney function before starting these medicines to make sure the person's kidneys are working normally. The doctor will also review other medicines before prescribing these medicines and may choose to adjust some of the other medicines while starting SGLT2 inhibitors. Once the doctor has determined the right dose, the person should take these medicines as prescribed. Most people take this medicine once a day by mouth. These medicines should be taken preferably at the same time each day.

Do not run out of this medicine; plan to call ahead and get refills.

After a missed dose, the person can take it within two or three hours. However, if it is almost time for the next dose, skip the missed dose and resume the regular schedule. Under no circumstances should you double the dose to make up for the missed one.

How to Stop the Medicine

SGLT2 inhibitors should be stopped only under the guidance of a doctor, even if they are not working or are causing side effects. She may choose to add other medicines while SGLT2 inhibitors are being stopped.

Who Should Avoid SGLT2 Inhibitors?

People with these problems should avoid or be cautious with SGLT2 inhibitors:

- kidney problems or
- increased disposition to infection.

People using other diabetes medicines as well as other diuretics should check with their physician while SGLT2 inhibitors are being started. The doctor may choose to decrease the dose of those medicines while SGLT2 inhibitors are being started.

Eight

YOUR TEAMMATES WITHIN THE HEALTH CARE SYSTEM

I felt that everyone was blowing me off; their answers were vague. But once I knew what questions to ask whom, I got all the information I needed. Now, I am more confident that I am doing the right thing.

—*Amy, whose parent has advanced heart disease*

Heart care is a team endeavor. This team is made up of many members from the health care system, but the person is the captain, and you are the vice-captain. To get the best results, it is important to understand your teammates, their background, and their expertise. Based on this information, the right questions, requests, and concerns can be directed to the right expert to get responses based on their experience and knowledge. This will help you understand the person's medical condition and ways to improve it. On the other hand, a question directed to someone without the requisite expertise will lead to frustrating, vague information at best and misinformation at worst.

So let us dive in to understand your teammates, their roles, and the right questions pertaining to their expertise.

HEALTH CARE TEAM IN THE HOSPITAL SETTING

Cardiologist

For people hospitalized for heart problems, the cardiologist directs the person's care. After four years of medical school, the cardiologist spends three years of training in internal medicine followed by three years of training as a cardiologist. The cardiologist may recruit help from colleagues such as:

- **Heart failure specialist:** A cardiologist with an additional one or more years of training in heart failure, left ventricular assist devices (LVADs), and heart transplantation.

- **Interventional cardiologist:** A cardiologist with an additional two years of training to perform angioplasties, place stents, and conduct other procedures.
- **Electrophysiologist:** A cardiologist with an additional two years of training in managing heart rhythm problems with medicines and complex procedures such as pacemakers, implantable cardioverter defibrillators, and ablation.
- **Cardiac surgeon:** Depending on the person's individual needs, a cardiac surgeon may also be involved in the person's care. For people hospitalized with the sole purpose of surgery, the surgeon directs the person's care. In other cases, the surgeon consults if the cardiologist believes that cardiac surgery will benefit the person. Beyond the four years of medical school, cardiac surgeons spend another five years in general surgical training followed by two or three years of specialized training in cardiac surgery. All of them perform coronary artery bypass grafting and valve surgeries, but depending on their experience, they may or may not perform LVAD surgery and heart transplantation. If the person needs an LVAD or heart transplantation, he may be referred to the surgeon with expertise in it.

What Questions Are Appropriate to Ask the Cardiologist?

- What is the person's diagnosis?
- Are alternative diagnoses being considered?
- How will the condition be treated?
- What tests will be performed today?
- What do we do if the test is positive? What if it is negative?
- What new medicine is going to be started?
- What are its major side effects?
- Does it replace another medicine?
- What procedure will be done today?
- How is it done?
- Are there alternatives to the procedure?
- Will this procedure prolong the person's life? Will it relieve symptoms?
- Who will do the procedure? May I talk with her?
- What are the complications of the procedure?
- How long will the person be hospitalized?
- Will other physicians be involved in the person's care?

Hospitalist

For people with complex medical problems, a hospitalist may play the primary role in the person's care, leaving the cardiologist to focus on heart-related issues. The hospitalist collaborates and coordinates care between specialists while the person is admitted to the hospital. Beyond four years of medical school, hospitalists spend three years of training in internal medicine.

What Questions are Appropriate for the Hospitalist?

- What is the primary diagnosis?
- Are alternative diagnoses being considered? How can the condition be treated?
- Are other organs affected?
- Do we need to involve specialists in that field?
- Will you coordinate the communication between specialists?
- Are there conflicting recommendations from specialists?
- How do we resolve them?
- Who will decide on release from the hospital?
- How is the person progressing on a day-to-day basis?
- What tests will be performed today?
- What do we do if the test is positive? What if it is negative?
- Is a new medicine going to be started?
- What are the major side effects?
- Does it replace another medicine?
- How long will the person be hospitalized?
- Does the person need outpatient physical therapy? Cardiac rehab?

Nurse Practitioner

Nurse practitioners have basic training and registration as a nurse with a four-year undergraduate degree and an advanced master's degree. Under the supervision of a physician, they take a detailed history, perform a physical exam, and provide day-to-day treatment while the person is hospitalized. Many of them have years of experience in the field and can be a great source of information.

If a nurse practitioner checks on the person daily, she may be a great source of reliable information about the tests, treatments and their side effects, complications, and alternatives. She will help coordinate care of the person with other team members in and out of the hospital. They are aware of community resources useful to people and their caregivers. They have greater time flexibility than physicians, and directing clinical questions to them will generally yield satisfactory responses.

What Questions Are Appropriate for Nurse Practitioners?

- How is the person doing compared with yesterday?
- What were the results of the tests performed yesterday?
- What changes will be made to the person's medicines today?
- We did not understand something that the doctor said. Can you explain it to us?
- Are any procedures planned for today?
- If so, can you explain the procedure?
- How will it help the person?
- Are there alternatives?
- Will the person be under anesthesia?
- How long does it generally take?
- Will any medicines be changed before the test?
- What time do you think the doctor will see the person?
- What is your estimate as to when the person can be discharged?

During discharge, ask:

- Can we go over the medicine list?
- Can we go over the need for these new medicines?
- What activities can the person safely perform at home?
- Is the person safe at home? Will he be able to manage daily activities?
- When will the person visit the clinic after the hospital stay?
- Can the person get a work excuse for this hospital stay?
- How can the person prevent future admissions?
- What precautions should the person take at home?
- What ominous signs should trigger us to contact the doctor's office?

Physician Assistant

Physician assistants, like nurse practitioners, have a graduate degree and certification. They work in similar capacity to nurse practitioners. If a physician assistant to the cardiologist is involved in the person's care, she will have similar expertise as a nurse practitioner. Also, many physician assistants work with and assist surgeons during surgeries and may be able to carry out minor procedures independently.

Nurse

Registered nurses (RNs) have either an associate's degree or four-year undergraduate degree in nursing. In the hospital, they provide hands-on person care, coordinate tests and treatments prescribed by the doctor, dispense medicines, and offer education, advice, and emotional support to people and caregivers. They watch for the person's progress on an hour-to-hour basis and inform the doctor of any worrisome signs or symptoms. They supervise licensed practical nurses (LPNs) to help the person.

Nurses work in eight- or twelve-hour shifts and are responsible for three to six patients in the hospital. Although hospitals try to provide the same nurse every day, it may not be possible considering scheduling conflicts and workload. When nurses change shifts, they perform an official handoff to the incoming nurse. Caregivers can request a bedside handoff to ensure that everyone agrees on the person's situation, progress, and outlook.

What Questions Are Appropriate for Nurses?

- Can the person have something for pain?
- When will the person have the radiograph, magnetic resonance imaging scan, or computed tomography scan that the doctor ordered?
- What are the side effects of this medicine?
- Is the person supposed to take a higher dose of medicine? He takes a much lower dose at home.
- When can the person eat?
- Can the person sit up in a chair?
- Can the person go for a walk?
- When will the physical therapist or occupational therapist see the person today?
- We would like to talk to a chaplain. Can you arrange it?
- Can the social worker or case manager explain the insurance situation to us?

Licensed Practical Nurses (LPNs)

LPNs get one year of training at a technical or community college and then pass a certification exam. LPNs are trained in basic nursing care (e.g., checking blood pressure and temperature, inserting catheters). They help the person in daily activities (e.g., bathing, dressing). They can train caregivers in performing some of these activities at home. Caregivers should let the LPNs know what they have learned while helping the person with daily activities at home.

What Questions Are Appropriate for the LPN?

- Can you help the person sit up, eat, or go to the bathroom?
- The intravenous line is beeping. Can you please do something about it?
- The person's electrocardiogram alarms are beeping. Can you do something about it?
- What was the person's blood pressure today? Temperature?
- The person is in pain. Can you ask the nurse to come in?

Pharmacist

Pharmacists undergo two or four years of undergraduate training followed by four years of training to earn a doctor of pharmacy degree. Pharmacists are experts in medicines and their doses, effects, side effects, and medicine interactions. They ensure that home medicines are correctly recorded in the hospital system and will inform the doctors if any new prescription interacts with the other medicines the person takes. Pharmacists also offer unbiased opinions on the efficacy of medicines new to the market. If unusual symptoms occur after a new medicine is started, the pharmacist will offer the team insight into potential rare side effects of medicines.

Some hospitals have clinical pharmacists who participate directly with the team and offer input on any new medicine the team is considering.

What Questions Are Appropriate for a Pharmacist?

- When should the person take this medicine? Before breakfast or after? Does it have to be taken with food?
- Will it interact with any other medicine?
- What are the main side effects of the new medicine we need to look for?
- How should these medicines be stored?
- The person has the same medicine at home in a higher dose. Can he take just half of it?

- Are there cheaper alternatives to this medicine?
- Will this medicine interact with food? What food items should the person avoid?
- Will this medicine interact with supplements?

Social Worker

A social worker has four years of undergraduate training in social work. Some social workers go on to earn a graduate degree in different fields of social work.

Illness and hospitalizations can be stressful, and decision-making in the hospital can cause further stress for the people and caregivers. Social workers understand the emotional burdens that disease places on the person and caregiver and work with the family to alleviate them. In the hospital, social workers help the person and caregivers navigate the health care system, services, and resources in the hospital and community.

They understand and help navigate the complexities of the financial issues related to hospitalization. Social workers can help coordinate home health nurses, physical therapists, occupational therapists, and speech therapists. They also coordinate transportation to doctor's visits after release from the hospital. Social workers can be a good resource for discussing health care directives and understanding the nuances of different options. Social workers act as patient advocates and facilitate communication between people, caregivers, and the health care team.

What Questions Are Appropriate for a Social Worker?

- I am not sure if the person is depressed or anxious and what to do about it. Can you help?
- The person does not want to undergo this surgery but is not able to talk to the doctor about it. Can you help?
- Is this new procedure covered by the person's insurance?
- Will insurance pay for these medicines?
- The person wants to change his health care proxy and advanced directive. Can you help us with it?
- Culturally, we are opposed to this procedure due to our beliefs. How can we communicate with the doctor?

Case Manager

Case managers have an undergraduate degree in sociology, health policy, or social justice. The prime responsibilities of a case manager are to coordinate the care of the person and help him transition from the hospital to home.

A case manager generally meets with the person and caregiver to understand and meet the person's needs. Case managers help people find the right nursing home, skilled nursing facility, or rehabilitation facility after hospital release. They can help coordinate at-home care (e.g., nurses, physical therapist, occupational therapist, speech therapist). Case managers have some overlapping responsibilities with social workers.

What Questions Are Appropriate for Case Managers?

- Who will administer intravenous medicine at home?
- Can a physical, occupational, or speech therapist provide treatment at home?
- Can the person go to a short-term nursing facility close to my home?
- Can the person be placed in a nursing home?
- I am not sure I can help with bathing, dressing, or other activities. Can someone come home and help him?
- Is there a support group that we can join?

Dietitian

Dieticians are trained nutrition professionals with at least four years of undergraduate training in a certified, accredited program and the requisite practicum training in addition to passing a certification exam. In the hospital, a registered dietitian can educate the person and caregiver about nutrition and provide medical nutrition therapy. They are also responsible for food service operations.

What Questions Are Appropriate for a Dietitian?

- The person is on a heart-healthy diet, but he does not like particular foods. Can we replace them with something else?
- The doctors talk about low salt. Can you explain how we can eliminate salt from the diet?
- The pharmacist told us that something interacts with the person's medicines and that he should avoid it. What can I replace it with?

- How can we count calories?
- How can we follow the fluid restrictions?
- What is a heart-healthy diet?
- How can we get more fruits and vegetables in the diet when he is such a picky eater?
- The doctor wants the person to lose weight. What kind of diet will help him achieve that?
- Do you think that the South Beach, keto, or paleo diet will help him?
- We are trying to cut out meat. What are high-protein alternatives?
- The doctor mentioned the high-fiber diet. What is it?
- He has a poor appetite. Can you suggest how to keep him well nourished?

Physical Therapist

A physical therapist is a trained professional who has completed three years of doctorate-level training in physical therapy education after four years of undergraduate training. They also must pass a certification exam. Some of them complete residency training programs and/or fellowship training in a specific field. They work with the person to restore physical function, improve mobility, relieve pain, and limit or prevent physical disabilities after an injury or illness. They also maintain and promote fitness and health.

In the hospital, once the doctor deems it safe, the person starts working with a physical therapist to increase their activities. They may start by sitting up in bed and progress to walking up and down the stairs before being released from the hospital. In the hospital, the physical therapist ensures that the person can function adequately to be safe at home. Often physical therapy is continued on an outpatient basis for as long as six weeks.

What Questions Are Appropriate for a Physical Therapist?

- What is the person's level of function?
- How is he progressing?
- What are his mobility goals before release?
- Is the person safe to go home?
- In which aspects of daily life will the person need help? How much help will be needed?
- If he is not safe to go home, should we consider a rehabilitation facility? A nursing home?
- Does the person need training to prevent falls?

- What exercises should the person do at home to improve function and mobility? To improve range of motion? To improve balance?
- What kind of help can you provide?

Occupational Therapist

An occupational therapist has four years of undergraduate training in occupational therapy. Most have a graduate degree obtained over two and a half years after college or a doctorate in occupational therapy obtained over three years after college.

An occupational therapist works with the person in the hospital to facilitate return to daily activities in his environment, whether it is at home or a nursing home. An occupational therapist interviews the person and caregiver in the hospital to understand the person's health, abilities, and home environment and your abilities. The therapist also understands which activities the person wishes to perform and why.

The therapist suggests modifications in activities so that the person can perform them independently or with minimal help. She may also recommend use of aids, equipment, or tools to facilitate these activities. The therapist may also recommend a change in environment to improve the person's ability to function (e.g., chair lift, hospital bed at home). They work with you to recognize how much help is needed, keeping the person's limitations in mind.

What Questions Are Appropriate for an Occupational Therapist?

- What can the person and I do to get back to a normal life? What activities should we do at home?
- Would you recommend alternative therapy (e.g., massage therapy) to help the person progress?
- Does the person need any equipment at home to perform routine activities?
- What help can you provide to facilitate the person's progress?
- What changes can we make at home to help the person?

Respiratory Therapist

Respiratory therapists complete a two-year associate's degree or four-year bachelor's degree program and then pass a certification test.

In the hospital, a respiratory therapist helps manage ventilators, administer nebulizers (breathing treatments), perform blood draws and analyze samples to check blood oxygen levels, and manage artificial airways.

What Questions Are Appropriate for a Respiratory Therapist?

- How long will the person continue to be on a ventilator?
- Are there alternatives to a ventilator?
- What is the blood oxygen level? Does he need to be treated for it?

As you have noticed, care of the person in the hospital is a team endeavor, with many team members with a range of training, experience, and expertise. Other teammates might be involved in the person's care, depending on his unique situation. Asking the right questions of the right expert will help obtain the information needed to continue the person's progress and provide a seamless transition between the hospital and home.

HEALTH CARE TEAM IN THE OUTPATIENT SETTING

Nurse

In the doctor's office, a nurse is responsible for coordinating multiple aspects of the person's care. The nurse is the point of contact for the person and the caregiver. She keeps open the communication line between the person, caregiver, and physician. The nurse can also advise the person about nutrition, medicines, pain management, and keeping track of blood pressure, heart rate, and weight. She is the point of contact for you for any concerning signs or symptoms.

When the doctor orders a test, the nurse will explain where and when to show up for it. She receives the results and passes it on to the doctor. Based on the doctor's assessment and recommendations, she will communicate the next steps in care to the person and family. She also calls in prescriptions and refills as needed. If the doctor requests a procedure or surgery, the nurse explains the procedure, what to expect from it, where and when to show up, which medicines to stop before the procedure, and care to be taken before the procedure.

When the person visits the doctor, a nurse gets necessary information before the doctor comes into the room. She may check the person's vital signs, review medicines, and ask about symptoms. Alternatively, she supervises a nurse assistant who may be assigned this role.

What Questions Are Appropriate for a Nurse?

- When is the person's test?
- Where should the person go for surgery?
- Does the person need to stop any medicines before surgery?
- Did the person's test results come in? Has the doctor looked at them?
- The person has a fever and slight cough. Should we worry?
- The person's heart rate is 130 beats a minute. Does he need to see the doctor?
- The person needs a prescription refill. Could you call in a refill for medicine X?
- Are there any dietary restrictions?
- The doctor mentioned that the person needs to see a lung doctor. Has that appointment been made?

Nurse Practitioner and Physician Assistant

In the outpatient setting, the nurse practitioner and physician assistant play an important role in the care of a person with heart disease. They see people for routine visits and answer questions. It is not uncommon for a person to see a nurse practitioner for six months or more with no contact with the doctor.

However, the doctor supervises the work of the nurse practitioner and physician assistant. If there are any new symptoms or concerns, the doctor is consulted by these advanced practice providers. The person and family should direct all health-related questions to them.

What Questions Are Appropriate for a Nurse Practitioner or Physician Assistant?

- How is the person's heart functioning?
- When will the person have his next echocardiogram?
- Why does the person need to do the test?
- Why does the person need the procedure?
- Can you explain the benefits of the procedure?
- What is the advantage of the medicine?
- Is there a generic alternative to the medicine?

Device Clinic

A device clinic staffs a team specialized in the care of people with implanted heart devices such as pacemakers and implantable cardioverter defibrillators. They monitor the device and problems with the device and the electrical system of the heart registered by the device.

Typically, this team checks the device on a home monitoring system or in the clinic every three to six months. They also receive alerts about any abnormalities registered on the device.

When the person is assessed in the device clinic, a nurse or a technician uses a laptop-like gadget to communicate with the implanted device. She checks the information stored in the device and tests the device to ensure proper functioning.

The person's device can be monitored from home using a home monitoring system. Device clinic staff will perform routine checks of the device through this home monitor. This staff is the best resource for education on the devices.

What Questions Are Appropriate for Device Clinic Staff?

- How much battery life does the person's pacemaker or implantable cardioverter defibrillator have?
- The person felt palpitations yesterday. Did his device register anything?
- Did the person have atrial fibrillation recently?
- Is the device working well?
- When is the next device check? In the clinic or from home?

INTERACTING WITH THE HEALTH CARE TEAM

You have a wealth of knowledge and insight. The health care team understands the unique needs of the person with the help of you and helps you understand the person's heart disease, medicines, and warning signs. You are the link between everyday life at home and the health care system.

Effective caregivers learn to interact and communicate proficiently with the health care team. This can be best accomplished if you know the roles and expertise of the team members.

First and foremost, you should identify the key health care professionals in the person's care. By recognizing their background and expertise, you will be able to direct questions to the appropriate person. On the other hand, asking a team member a question outside the scope of their expertise will create confusion and frustration for everyone.

The next step is to keep all the information about the person organized. It is important to create a print or electronic person folder to keep all critical information in one location. Keeping an electronic record will ensure that you can access it from anywhere. If you choose to have a paper copy, keep it in a location easily accessible, even in an emergency.

The following information should be included in the person's folder:

- person's medical history;
- diagnosis (e.g., diabetes, kidney disease);
- past surgeries (gallbladder removal, bypass surgery);
- past or current use of tobacco, alcohol, or street medicines;
- health care team;

Primary care physician	Dr. Johnson	xxx-xxx-xxxx
Cardiologist	Dr. Smith	xxx-xxx-xxxx
Pharmacy	Greenmart	xxx-xxx-xxxx
Home care agency		

- allergies (e.g., penicillin causes a rash);
- medicine list;
- current medicines;

Medicine	Dose	Date started	Reason for taking	Side effects/ notes
Metoprolol	25 mg twice a day	12/12/2012	Heart disease	

- supplements or over-the-counter medicines;
- past medicines;

Medicine	Dose	Date started	Date stopped	Notes
Diltiazem	120 mg once a day	5/6/2006	12/12/2012	Replaced with metoprolol

- implantable cardioverter defibrillator, pacemaker, or loop recorder;
- brand;
- implanted on;
- phone number for pacemaker clinic;

Date	Weight	Blood pressure	Heart rate	Short of breath?	Foot or leg swelling or abdomen bloating?	How do you feel? Other symptoms?
				Yes/No	Yes/No	
				Yes/No	Yes/No	
				Yes/No	Yes/No	
				Yes/No	Yes/No	
				Yes/No	Yes/No	
				Yes/No	Yes/No	

- photocopy of the person's insurance card, Medicare card, prescription coverage plan, long-term care insurance card, and dental and vision insurance cards; and
- legal documents (e.g., living will or advanced care directive, durable power of attorney for health care or health care proxy, physician's order for life-sustaining treatment).

The next step in being an effective caregiver is to be the spokesperson for the person. It is critical for you to attend the person's appointments with doctors, nurse practitioners, and other health care providers. Having another pair of ears will help the person better understand and remember the information. You may also consider taking notes to aid memory later.

In addition to the person's folder, you should bring this list to all visits:

My questions for this visit with [insert doctor name], in the order of importance, are:

1. _____

2. _____

3. _____

4. _____

5. _____

During these discussions, when a test is suggested, gather this information about it:

- What is the test?
- Is it an invasive procedure?
- What happens if the test is abnormal?
- What happens if the test is normal?
- What happens if the person does not do this test?
- What bad outcomes can we expect from this test?
- What are the risks of the test?
- What are the benefits?
- Will it change the outcome of the disease or the person's lifestyle?

When medicines, procedures, or surgeries are suggested, ask these questions:

- What is the medicine, procedure, or surgery?
- What are the side effects? Complications?
- What will successful intervention do? Will it improve longevity or improve symptoms in cases like this?
- What happens if the person decides not to undergo this treatment? Is there an alternative?
- Considering the person's goals and other conditions, is it reasonable to consider this choice?
- How long is the recovery period? What kind of help will be required during the recovery?
- Will the person return home after recovering from the surgery?

For specific tests/procedures, refer to chapter 5.

Emergency Department Visits

Visits to the emergency department are not uncommon for people with heart disease. If you notice frequent visits, you should keep a kit ready to be prepared to participate in care while the person is in the emergency department.

Keep a copy of the updated person folder mentioned previously, complete with the person's medical history, medicines, insurance information, and legal documents. Keep papers and a pen ready for taking notes. Some caregivers have suggested having cash, bottled water, healthy snacks, puzzles, or reading material ready. A change of clothes for the person may also be helpful to have in this kit.

Hospitalization

When the person is hospitalized, you may feel that your caregiving role has been suspended. Some caregivers take the opportunity to take a respite. Although this may be reasonable in some cases, in general, caregivers should stay involved in the care of the person while he is in the hospital. Over time, caregivers develop expertise in the person's priorities, preferences, and needs at home and can communicate them to the health care team. Caregivers can further help during the person's hospital stay by:

- ensuring that the team knows the person's medical history, allergies, and medicines;
- helping hospital caretakers understand how the person prefers to shower, sleep, and eat; and
- helping the caretakers understand the person's preferences for help in daily activities.

In the hospital, the team does not remain constant. The nursing staff and nurse assistants change from morning to evening. The doctors may change from one day to the next, and new consultants are asked to offer input. Thus, you may be the only continuity throughout the hospitalization to ensure that the person continues to progress steadily. You can effectively play this role by:

- Participating in the nursing change-of-shift report so that you understand which major issues are being addressed and what safety concerns get passed on from one nursing shift to another: You should bring up any concerns not raised so that either the omission can be corrected or you can be given an explanation for why it is no longer a concern.

- Participating in team rounds: Each morning, the health care team goes to each person's bedside, and the nurse presents information to a team of doctors, social workers, physical therapists, counselors, and nurse managers. The team discusses new concerns that have come up, any progress in the person's health, input from consultants, new medicines to be added, any tests to be performed, and the plan for release. Participating in these rounds will help you understand the plan for the day and the progress toward hospital release. It is also an opportunity to ask questions and raise concerns.
- Being aware of the current medicines being given in the hospital: Medicine errors are not uncommon in hospitals. Wrong medicines and wrong doses are more common than one would like to believe. You can help prevent errors in medicine administration by keeping track of the medicines the patient is taking at home and what changes are being made in the hospital on a day-to-day basis. The pharmacists and/or the nurse can be your ally in this regard.
- Participating in the decision-making process by understanding which tests and treatment options are being suggested, asking questions (see relevant chapters for more information), and seeing whether it is in keeping with the person's wishes.
- Being aware of the consultant's recommendations and making sense of how they tie into the person's overall condition.

A hospital stay is also a good time to learn alternative and, in some cases, better ways to care for the person's daily needs from the professionals. Observing the way an experienced nurse assistant bathes the person, a nurse changes the dressing, and the physical therapist motivates the person will help you give better care at home.

Release from the Hospital

When the person is being released from the hospital, you play an important role in understanding the instructions so as to safely transition from the hospital to home. You should have a clear understanding of the following:

- What has been accomplished through this hospital admission?
- How can a future admission be prevented?
- What medicines have been discontinued? Why?
- What new medicines have been added? What do they do?

- What is the new list of medicines? Can we have prescriptions for those medicines?
- Are other blood tests, radiographs, or cardiac tests to be performed?
- When is the next office visit with the cardiologist?
- When is the next office visit with the primary care physician?
- Is any other consultation needed?
- Any special precautions that need to be taken?
- What warning signs should I look for?
- Any dietary or activity changes to be made after hospital release?
- When can the person resume normal activities? Exercise?
- Is cardiac rehab needed after release?

THE PALLIATIVE CARE TEAM

What Is Palliative Care?

Palliative care is the care of people with a serious medical condition in which the focus is improved quality of life through relief from stress and disease symptoms. A palliative care team consists of a doctor, nurse, social worker, chaplain, physical therapist, occupational therapist, dietitian, and psychologist. These specialists take a holistic approach to improve the quality of life of both the person and her family.

These teams offer care in all settings, such as hospitals, homes, or nursing homes. They may provide information and help the person create a plan based on her preferences. The palliative care team works together to address the physical, psychological, social, and spiritual needs of the person and caregivers. They help the person work on their advanced directives. The specialists help navigate the system with the multitude of health care providers with whom people with complex cardiac conditions interact. They can also facilitate communication between different health care teams. People enrolled in palliative care are appropriately referred to hospice care and derive great benefits from this timely referral.

The team can help with the emotional care of you and loved ones in addition to the person and can offer respite care. They may also help review advance care plans on an ongoing basis.

Studies have shown that when a palliative care team is involved, people spend less time in the hospital, are more satisfied with their care, and often die at home, if they so wish. Interestingly, they also live longer and have lower costs of care.

What Is the Role of Palliative Care and Hospice in Heart Failure?

Palliative care is recommended when people have a serious health condition. In people with heart failure, palliative care focuses on easing symptoms of shortness of breath, fatigue, and nausea.

If heart failure progresses, the current treatment is not working, and no other options are available, the doctor may recommend hospice care, which is specialized care for terminally ill people. The hospice care team consists of nurses, social workers, and volunteers who work with caregivers, family, and friends to provide comfort and care at home or in a specialized setting. The team focuses on providing physical, emotional, psychological, and spiritual support to the person, caregivers, friends, and family.

Is the Person Currently a Candidate for Palliative Care?

Palliative care can be used at all stages of illness, even when the expected life span is measured in years or decades. However, in general, it is most helpful when the person is at an advanced stage of disease.

People typically enroll in palliative care when they notice fatigue, shortness of breath, or chest pain with activities of daily living such as bathing, cooking, and getting dressed. People who are hospitalized often or getting multiple ICD shocks may also be considered for palliative care. In rare cases, emotional distress in people or their caregivers may be significant enough to use palliative services.

People receiving palliative care continue to receive all treatments necessary to improve and reverse the impact of the illness. You can discuss palliative care when the team thinks that the person may benefit from this expertise.

What Are the Benefits of Palliative Care?

High-quality palliative care can make the difference between a comfortable existence and suffering. Palliative care teams help decrease hospital stays, needless suffering through hospitalization, and decrease the costs of care. Palliative care also can help you and other family members with grief and bereavement.

What Questions Are Appropriate for the Palliative Care Team?

- The person has back pain, and the doctor says he cannot give any medicines safely. Can you help?

- What is a do-not-resuscitate order? What is an advance health directive?
- Should the person enroll in hospice?
- Is the new surgery being recommended right for the person at this stage of heart disease?
- Can you help the person change his power of attorney?
- As a caregiver, I am going through anxiety about the person's illness. What should I do?
- I do not feel capable of helping the person with daily activities. Can I get some help?
- Is the person dying?
- The person wants to be an organ donor. How do we document that?

What Is Hospice Care?

When the person makes a transition in their health care priority from increased survival with curative treatment to focusing on quality of life by way of relief from symptoms, the hospice care team gets involved. In general, at this stage, people have chosen to forego hospitalization and are focused on symptom relief at home.

People are referred to hospice care when their expected life span is less than six months. This team provides comfort and support to people and their families. Like a palliative care team, a hospice care team includes a doctor, nurse, social worker, chaplain, physical therapist, occupational therapist, dietitian, and psychologist.

It may be appropriate to start a discussion about hospice care if the person:

- is hospitalized frequently,
- is fatigued and out of breath at rest,
- depends on others for activities of daily living,
- is losing weight,
- has a stroke, or
- has multiple ICD shocks despite ablation procedures or is not a candidate for ablation.

What Services Can Hospice Care Provide?

- Home health aides to help with bathing, grooming, eating, and other personal health needs;
- trained volunteers who provide support services such as respite care, running errands, and preparing meals;

- bereavement support and counseling for caregivers and families;
- physical and occupational therapy to help the person develop new ways to perform daily tasks such as dressing, taking a shower, and moving safely around the house; and
- help with insurance, legal documents, and other practical issues.

You should ask the hospice team whether the person should continue medicines such as angiotensin-converting enzyme inhibitors or beta blockers.

When people are referred to hospice care appropriately, there is improved person and family satisfaction and understanding of expectations at the end of life, greater confidence in caring for the person at home, and improved ability to coordinate care. Hospice services can support you and the rest of the family through the final stages of the person's life and grief after the person's death.

Nine

USEFUL INFORMATION TO HAVE ON HAND: RECORDING SHEETS

The first year was tough; he had to be admitted four times. Medicines were changed many times. Now he is back to good health. He works a full-time job. I hardly have to do anything. He takes his medicines, and that is it, but I tell you, it was a lot of hard work for a long time.

—*Jennifer, whose father has heart disease*

It can be especially challenging communicating your concerns to health care providers when caring for a person with advanced heart disease.

The following pages are for you to fill out before you call or see a health care provider. You may wish to remove them from this book or, better yet, make multiple photocopies. By gathering this information in advance, you'll likely find the call or visit more productive and helpful.

INFORMATION TO GATHER BEFORE CALLING A HEALTH CARE PROVIDER

This form can help you organize and communicate a new concern to the health care provider. It is especially useful if there are multiple caregivers sharing responsibilities.

Name: _____

DOB: _____

Primary care physician: _____

Primary cardiologist: _____

Nurse you usually talk to: _____

Cardiac diseases: _____

Previous surgeries: _____

List of current medicines: _____

What are the symptoms of concern? _____

How long has this been going on? _____

How do the symptoms start? _____

How long do the symptoms last? _____

What makes the symptoms better? _____

What makes the symptoms worse? _____

Any other associated symptoms? _____

Has this happened before and, if so, what did the doctors do? _____

_____

Have there been any recent changes in medicines? _____

Has there been a recent change in diet? _____

Current weight? _____

Average weight? _____

Heart rate and blood pressure? _____

Has the person been admitted to the hospital or visited the emergency
room in the last twelve months? _____

PERSONAL HEALTH RECORD

This form is a handy record of the person's family contacts, physicians, medical problems, medicines, allergies, and insurance. Almost all visits to the
health care team require some or all this information.

Name: _____

DOB: _____

Power of attorney: _____

Living will: Yes/No _____

Family contact and phone: _____

Insurance: _____

Medical history: _____

_____

_____

Diagnosis (e.g., diabetes):

- _____

- _____

- _____

Previous surgery with date:

- _____

- _____

- _____

Past or current use of tobacco, alcohol, or street medicines:

- _____

- _____

- _____

HEALTH CARE TEAM

	Name	Phone Number
Primary care physician:		
Cardiologist:		
Pharmacy:		
Home care agency:		

ALLERGIES (e.g., penicillin causes a rash)

Medicinal/Chemical	Reaction

CURRENT MEDICINES

Medicine	Dose	Date started	Reason for taking	Side effects/ notes

Supplements or over-the-counter medicines:

- _____
- _____
- _____

PAST MEDICINES

Medicine	Dose	Date started	Reason for taking	Side effects/ notes

Implantable cardioverter defibrillator, pacemaker, or loop recorder:

- Brand: _____
- Implanted on: _____
- Phone number for pacemaker clinic: _____

My observations of concern are:

1. Energy: _____

2. Diet: _____

3. Hospital visits: _____

4. Medication effect: _____

My questions for this visit with [insert doctor name], in the order of importance, are:

1. _____

2. _____

3. _____

4. _____

5. _____

VITAL SIGNS RECORDING SHEET

Use this sheet to record the person's vital signs regularly so that you'll get to know their usual measurements. Bring this sheet with you during provider visits and make additional copies for future use.

Date	Weight	Blood pressure	Heart rate	Short of breath?	Foot or leg swelling or abdomen bloating?	How do you feel? Other symptoms?
				Yes/No	Yes/No	
				Yes/No	Yes/No	
				Yes/No	Yes/No	
				Yes/No	Yes/No	
				Yes/No	Yes/No	
				Yes/No	Yes/No	

NOTES

CHAPTER 5:
COMMON HEART CONDITIONS, TESTS, AND TREATMENTS

1. Stephan Fihn et al., "2014 ACC/AHA/AATS/PCNA/SCAI/STS Focused Update of the Guideline for the Diagnosis and Management of People with Stable Ischemic Heart Disease: A Report of the American College of Cardiology/American Heart Association Task Force on Practice Guidelines, and the American Association for Thoracic Surgery, Preventive Cardiovascular Nurses Association, Society for Cardiovascular Angiography and Interventions, and Society of Thoracic Surgeons," *Circulation* 130, no. 19 (2014): 1749–67, doi: 10.1161/CIR.0000000000000095; Stephan Fihn et al., "2012 ACCF/AHA/ACP/AATS/PCNA/SCAI/STS Guideline for the Diagnosis and Management of Patients with Stable Ischemic Heart Disease: Executive Summary: A Report of the American College of Cardiology Foundation/American Heart Association task force on practice guidelines, and the American College of Physicians, American Association for Thoracic Surgery, Preventive Cardiovascular Nurses Association, Society for Cardiovascular Angiography and Interventions, and Society of Thoracic Surgeons," *Circulation* 126, no. 25 (2012): 3097–137, doi: 10.1161/CIR.0b013e3182776f83; Jerome Fleg et al., "Secondary Prevention of Atherosclerotic Cardiovascular Disease in Older Adults: A Scientific Statement from the American Heart Association," *Circulation* 128, no. 22 (2013): 2422–46, doi: 10.1161/01.cir.0000436752.99896.22.

2. Jerome Fleg et al., "Secondary Prevention."

CHAPTER 6:
DAY-TO-DAY CARE ISSUES

1. P. M. Ridker, P. Libby, and J. E. Buring, "Risk Markers and Primary Prevention of Coronary Heart Disease," in *Braunwald's Heart Disease: A Textbook of Cardiovascular Medicine*, 11th edition, ed. Douglas Zipes, Peter Libby, Robert Bonow, Douglas Mann, and Gordon Tomasell (Philadelphia, PA: Elsevier; 2019), chapter 45.

2. L. Djoussé and J. M. Gaziano, "Alcohol Consumption and Heart Failure: A Systematic Review," *Current Atherosclerosis Reports* 10, no. 2 (2008): 117–20.

3. Ridker, Libby, and Buring, "Risk Markers."

4. American College of Cardiology, "Despite Concerns, Caffeine Is OK for People with Heart Failure," CardioSmart, https://www.cardiosmart.org/News-and -Events/2016/10/Despite-Concerns-Caffeine-is-Safe-for-People-with-Heart-Failure (accessed May 16, 2019).

BIBLIOGRAPHY

American College of Cardiology. "Despite Concerns, Caffeine Is OK for People with Heart Failure." CardioSmart. Accessed May 16, 2019. https://www.cardio smart.org/News-and-Events/2016/10/Despite-Concerns-Caffeine-is-Safe-for -People-with-Heart-Failure.

Centers for Disease Control and Prevention. "Important Facts about Falls." National Center for Injury Prevention and Control, 2011. Last accessed May 23, 2021. http://www.cdc.gov/homeandrecreationalsafety/falls/adultfalls.html.

Djoussé, L., and J. M. Gaziano. "Alcohol Consumption and Heart Failure: A Systematic Review." *Current Atherosclerosis Reports* 10, no. 2 (2008): 117–20.

Fihn, Stephan, James C. Blankenship, Karen P. Alexander, John A. Bittl, John G. Byrne, Barbara J. Fletcher, Gregg C. Fonarow, Richard A. Lange, Glenn N. Levine, Thomas M. Maddox, Srihari S. Naidu, E. Magnus Ohman, and Peter K. Smith. "2014 ACC/AHA/AATS/PCNA/SCAI/STS Focused Update of the Guideline for the Diagnosis and Management of Patients with Stable Ischemic Heart Disease: A Report of the American College of Cardiology/American Heart Association Task Force on Practice Guidelines, and the American Association for Thoracic Surgery, Preventive Cardiovascular Nurses Association, Society for Cardiovascular Angiography and Interventions, and Society of Thoracic Surgeons." *Circulation* 130, no. 19 (2014): 1749–67. doi: 10.1161/CIR.0000000000000095.

Fihn, Stephan, Julius Gardin, Jonathan Abrams, Kathleen Berra, James Blankenship, Apostolos Dallas, Pamela Douglas, Joanne Foody, Thomas Gerber, Alan Hinderliter, Spencer King III, Paul Kligfield, Harlan Krumholz, Raymond Kwong, Michael Lim, Jane Linderbaum, Michael Mack, Mark Munger, Richard Prager, Joseph Sabik, Leslee Shaw, Joanna Sikkema, Craig Smith Jr., Sidney Smith Jr., John Spertus, Sankey Williams, American College of Cardiology Foundation. "2012 ACCF/AHA/ACP/AATS/PCNA/SCAI/STS Guideline for the Diagnosis and Management of Patients with Stable Ischemic Heart Disease: Executive Summary: A Report of the American College of Cardiology Foundation/American Heart Association Task Force on Practice Guidelines, and the American College of Physicians, American Association for Thoracic Surgery, Preventive

Cardiovascular Nurses Association, Society for Cardiovascular Angiography and Interventions, and Society of Thoracic Surgeons." *Circulation* 126, no. 25 (2012): 3097–137. doi: 10.1161/CIR.0b013e3182776f83.

Fleg, Jerome, Daniel Forman, Kathy Berra, Vera Bittner, James Blumenthal, Michael Chen, Susan Cheng, Dalane Kitzman, Mathew Maurer, Michael Rich, Win-Kuang Shen, Mark Williams, Susan Zieman, American Heart Association Committees on Older Populations and Exercise Cardiac Rehabilitation and Prevention of the Council on Clinical Cardiology, Council on Cardiovascular and Stroke Nursing, Council on Lifestyle and Cardiometabolic Health. "Secondary Prevention of Atherosclerotic Cardiovascular Disease in Older Adults: A Scientific Statement from the American Heart Association." *Circulation* 128, no. 22 (2013): 2422–46. Last accessed May 23, 2021. doi: 10.1161/01.cir.0000436752.99896.22.

Gibbons, Raymond, Gary Balady, J. Timothy Bricker, Bernard Chaitman, Gerald Fletcher, Victor Froelicher, Daniel B. Mark, Ben McCallister, Aryan Mooss, Michael O'Reilly, William Winters, Elliott Antman, Joseph Alpert, David Faxon, Valentin Fuster, Gabriel Gregoratos, Loren Hiratzka, Alice Jacobs, Richard Russell, Sidney Smith, American College of Cardiology/American Heart Association Task Force on Practice Guidelines, Committee to Update the 1997 Exercise Testing Guidelines. "ACC/AHA 2002 Guideline Update for Exercise Testing: A Report of the American College of Cardiology/American Heart Association Task Force on Practice Guidelines (Committee on Exercise Testing)." *Journal of the American College of Cardiology* 40, no. 8 (2002): 1531–40.

Kulik, Alexander, Marc Ruel, Hani Jneid, T. Bruce Ferguson, Loren Hiratzka, John Ikonomidis, Francisco Lopez-Jimenez, Sheila McNallan, Mahesh Patel, Véronique Roger, Frank Sellke, Domenic Sica, Lani Zimmerman, American Heart Association Council on Cardiovascular Surgery and Anesthesia. "Secondary Prevention after Coronary Artery Bypass Graft Surgery: A Scientific Statement from the American Heart Association." *Circulation* 131, no. 10 (2015): 927–64. Last accessed May 23, 2021. doi: 10.1161/CIR.0000000000000182.

Morrow, D. A., and J. A. de Lemos. "Stable Ischemic Heart Disease." In *Braunwald's Heart Disease: A Textbook of Cardiovascular Medicine*, 11th edition, ed. Douglas Zipes, Peter Libby, Robert Bonow, Douglas Mann, and Gordon Tomasell. Philadelphia, PA: Elsevier, 2019.

National Conference of State Legislatures. "Elderly Falls Prevention Legislation and Statutes." 2018. Last accessed May 23, 2021. http://www.ncsl.org/default .aspx?tabid=13854.

Nishimura, Rick, Catherine Otto, Robert Bonow, Blase Carabello, John Erwin III, Robert Guyton, Patrick O'Gara, Carlos Ruiz, Nikolaos Skubas, Paul Sorajja, Thoralf Sundt III, James Thomas, ACC/AHA Task Force Members. "2014 AHA/ACC

Guideline for the Management of Patients with Valvular Heart Disease: Executive Summary: A Report of the American College of Cardiology/American Heart Association Task Force on Practice Guidelines." *Journal of the American College of Cardiology* 63, no. 22 (2014): 2438–88. Last accessed May 23, 2021. doi: 10.1161/ CIR.0000000000000029.

Omer, S., L. D. Cornwell, and F. G. Bakaeen. "Acquired Heart Disease: Coronary Insufficiency." In *Sabiston Textbook of Surgery*, 20th edition, ed. C. M. Townsend Jr., R. D. Beauchamp, B. M. Evers, and K. L. Mattox. Philadelphia, PA: Elsevier, 2017.

Piña, Ileana, Carl Apstein, Gary Balady, Romualdo Belardinelli, Bernard Chaitman, Brian D. Duscha, Barbara Fletcher, Jerome Fleg, Jonathan Myers, Martin Sullivan, American Heart Association Committee on Exercise, Rehabilitation, and Prevention. "Exercise and Heart Failure: A Statement from the American Heart Association Committee on Exercise, Rehabilitation, and Prevention." *Circulation* 107 (2003): 1210–25.

Ridker, P. M., P. Libby, and J. E. Buring. "Risk Markers and Primary Prevention of Coronary Heart Disease." In *Braunwald's Heart Disease: A Textbook of Cardiovascular Medicine*, 11th edition, ed. Douglas Zipes, Peter Libby, Robert Bonow, Douglas Mann, and Gordon Tomasell (chapter 45). Philadelphia, PA: Elsevier, 2019.

Thompson, P. D., and P. A. Ades. "Exercise-Based, Comprehensive Cardiac Rehabilitation." In *Braunwald's Heart Disease: A Textbook of Cardiovascular Medicine*, 11th edition, ed. Douglas Zipes, Peter Libby, Robert Bonow, Douglas Mann, and Gordon Tomasell (chapter 54). Philadelphia, PA: Elsevier, 2019.

INDEX

warfarin, 176–179
  action, 176
  caution, 178–179
  interaction, 170, 177, 181, 185,
    191
  pregnancy, 179
  side effects, 176–177
    managing, 177
  surgery, 178
  use, 73, 122, 176

weight, 18, 26, 55, 144–146
  app, 138
  gain, 137
  ideal, 88, 137–138
Well Spouse Association, 44
Wheeze, 17

yoga, 135

Zaroxolyn. *See* metolazone

ABOUT THE AUTHOR

J Shah is a board-certified cardiologist and an epidemiologist. He was trained at Harvard Medical School and has practiced in various countries and diverse settings over the past twenty years. He is informed by best practices all across the globe and brings this vast experience to his patients' care. He hopes to empower patients and families with knowledge about their health and make them an integral part of their own health care team. He is passionate about patients' and the family's experience of health care and hopes to bring human elements back to medicine. When he is not seeing patients, he is writing, traveling, or hiking. He lives in Louisville, Kentucky.